Out of the Woods

To Law

ford

Matthew

Matthew & Lorraine Woods

chipmunkapublishing
the mental health publisher

All rights reserved, no part of this publication may be reproduced by any means, electronic, mechanical photocopying, documentary, film or in any other format without prior written permission of the publisher.

Published by

Chipmunkapublishing

PO Box 6872

Brentwood

Essex CM13 1ZT

United Kingdom

http://www.chipmunkapublishing.com

Copyright © Matthew Woods 2011

Edited by Nick Rainsford

Front cover photography courtesy of Claire Rivers

Inside artwork by Lorraine Woods

ISBN 978-1-84991-689-9

Chipmunkapublishing gratefully acknowledge the support of Arts Council England.

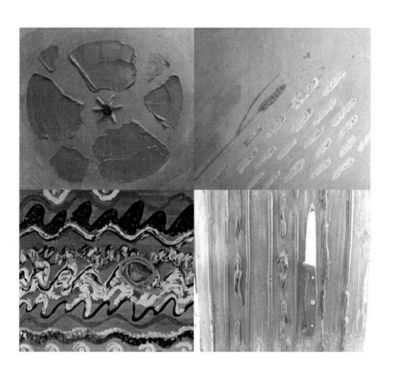

Matthew & Lorraine Woods

Dedicated to Sgt. Pilot Michael Warrick 1930-1953
Special thanks to Timi, Oliver Dachinger and Patrick
Duff for their care and contributions.

Matthew & Lorraine Woods

Chapter 1   Spectral Diversity

Chapter 2   Dandelion Clock

Chapter 3   Eternity Beach

Chapter 4   Name, Rank and Number

Chapter 5   Between the Candle and the Flame

Chapter 6   True Truant of Memories

Chapter 7   Enjoy Your Time in Passion's Eye

Chapter 8   Seeing the Wood For the Trees

Chapter 9   Parachute of Faith

Matthew & Lorraine Woods

Chapter 1 Spectral Diversity

Between the candle and the stars there was a story. They treated him with all the sins of society and its forefathers, the wax of his dreams, which changed to angel rain and began to fall in a deluge around him. They closed their curtains "Another challenge. Absolutely clear. When did your heart burn so frankly as this?" Through incomplete shedding, incomplete pain the silence was agitated- save the numb, cool space of winter. "I live in this odyssey watching the moon's gait backwards." Robed in white, majestic, so familiar, she hesitates and crosses the bridge. She is with me, has come to be with me. Would there be an impact of responsibility to do what we choose? If we practise choice, it has an effect on others and our relationships. With haste she sips the bitter gift and can't conceal her debonair- for how would this sweet maiden live without such innocence, she stoops and picks the bursting berry's blackest prime. Choices are with us each and every day. Perhaps in nature the ratio phi is used in varying complexities to map out life like a code? I believe that we all make choices according to spectral diversity- we all see things differently but have core realities in common, yet those cores can vary in strength depending on the degree of love accepted so far - the colours of the spectrum are understood differently and may be dependent on mood. No surprises please. How should I ensure there are none? Wisdom? Knowing that surprising things happen? I follow her down some stairs, her white dress flowing behind her. Spectral diversity is the binding factor, which creates colours for her life. Faster she runs but always a glimpse remaining. Down the spiral staircase, like a shell circling or a candle burning.

These stairs were the very stairs I stared up at as a 4 year old on my first day at school. Stairs leading to the age I would reach. Wooden spiral stairs, but this time, leading only downwards. Leading down to a basement, a huge vaulted basement, or sea cave. Of deep blue. Always at night. Angel'rain spoke "Perhaps the holy spirit in each one of us, laying resident in our hearts if we choose, causes the heart to govern the body as an ultimate source-centre. This connecting to God's pre-decision (in human term's) can give form to our whole existence and ensure a fulfilling journey through life; the whole starting point of good and bad may propel us to act and by consciously performing these actions, we realize consequences and move forward. In other words, the heart represents all our dynamism at the service of the mission that God has entrusted to us. Notions plucked from the heart, god infused, can place goodness and virtue in others lives. There is always good to be found if it is persued and like a chain reaction, the previous links form foundations for links to come.   Thoughts are wings of feathers for mankind who can never fly, and spectral diversity channelling plumes of thoughts may mean that we all perceive differently but all want to fly. We are not likely to know what it is to fly without aid while living on earth; there are some things that are just not meant to be. We can imagine by drawing on as many angles of experience relevant as possible to form an auto-reality but the truth is that it is not a real experience and is not likely to lead to the unexpected conclusions that can form new start points. Like a lie, a negative buzz is derived and even if good conclusion is reached, the buzz of assumption corrupts the idea and healthy mind. Psychosis buries heads with layered suppositions as these." The inquiring mind can be oh so foolish....

I replied; "The romance of flight has surrounded us since ancient myth- from Egypt come illustrations of winged gods, from Assyria, the winged bull, from Greece the winged horse, Pegasus and from Rome the god Mercury. We all see the world differently but have the same spectrum. The theory of spectral diversity. The Macedonian, Alexander the great, according to legend, journeyed to view the heavens in a chariot drawn by gryphons that were encouraged in this effort by pieces of meat placed just out of their reach. In England King Bladud is supposed to have attempted to fly over London in 852 BC but fell to his death. Oliver a Benedictine monk in 1026 jumped while fitted with wings from Malmesbury Abbey and after a short glide broke both his legs. The first successful Englishman to fly did so in his dreams." But the balloon was brought to the ground and no end of flipping the coins or scratching your initials in the arm of love could cut the braces of his desperation.

Unfortunately, the colour of her core was of a pale citrus, so on she searched for sure definition. She floated, for a long time, through the empty space, through dreams of string orchestras in sustained monotone. The murmured cloud, melting 'neath a marbled sky, the silence of her fear was diminishing but the respite of confluence with the soul told that dreams, even waking dreams, be chosen and unchosen? Did the baton conduct perfection or noise? Dreams are a picked daisy's prayer. She continued "That I was beautiful then, a taller kind under gravity of exposition. Let this remain in my stubborn memory. What am I, and what right has the influence of medication to make right of introspection? It ceased turmoil in the mind but at what cost? Picked vitality resting on rootless shores. I can only sustain moments and have not the energy to cry. Broken and deprived I am but a dream. Is it ok to dream but not to let your dreams become you? *For everything we are or seem, we are but a dream within a dream* (E Allen-Poe)". We have a need to lay our heads on a bed of reason and justification; an unriddling dream is a passage to that place of comfort.

As night turned to mystery, vole lay subject to the deepest redemption that a little soul had ever the pleasure of receiving. Thoughts of each bruise, misuse of drug, internal and external suffering came flooding. God saw to it that it would be undone that night. The pain was lifted or perhaps reversed, like a rebirth of man, a born again. Voles body twisted, turned, lifted, heaved, clamped, cajoled, and squeezed together to produce relief of past suffering that had always just been grasped in a dream. Vole focused his attention on prayer – God led him there. He lay on his homemade bed shared with a few fidgety beetles and flotsam moths and prayed, 'Come Holy Spirit, Come. Praise be to God. Thank you Father God. Please forgive me my sins. Come Holy Spirit, Come – Come rest within my body. Thank you Lord, Thank you Lord', and all the while Vole's body unravelled, the prayer continued.

And it was so. A series of several nights healing that vole fearlessly traversed with the love on his side. God penetrated Vole's mind as Mozart's Lacrimosa passionately stated its hope of rebirth for the first time. Vole, purified and restored looked toward another future in a dream. So we dreamt. Vampires roamed the land in secret covens searching for the apple of youth. A huge ray of fire had struck the ground. Out of this crater, a spiral tree emerged. In the gods, the penny colour of Iduna's eye led like an apple of youth fruiting along the dairy path. She was tricked under the influence of the vampires of the earth. She came to earth under the late summer moon, among the stone circles, in view of the meteor's crater. "Daughter to the stars chased the meteor's bloom, red setted with explosives where there is an apple of gold, thrown and crumpled to kinship".

As I saw her I was in rapture. The twinkling of the stars, love divine, together throughout time, crossed my path forever. She was precious to the gods and carried the secret of their youth in her casket of apples.

To a motion fingered by fermenting shells vampires crossed the oceans. As they swam into the night, aware of Iduna's laced casket, the moon shone down. They swooped down and stole the casket of apples from Iduna. The gods were angry and grew old.

I thought of my mortality, listening to the strange music of the vampires who were holding vigil there and thought that the most important things in life were the things that you got away with from the gods. A strange sensation gripped me, as if I was taken over by a malevolent force. I was aware that there was a realm beyond the senses in which we endure the elements of life. They put it down to the triumph of darkness over light as the dusk set in. This is a mixture of madness and innocence so close to us when we are young adults that the distance between it and the life centre inside us cannot be measured. The space between the candle and the flame. Through medication, age and coping strategies it has become something external, held further away from us every day like an unobtainable apple of youth. Like the darkness of the sound barrier, it's understanding is our very essence, since the snake tricked us under the pale moon in the Garden of Eden: the effects of that original sin are still being seen.

The age of innocence has long since gone
To bite at the nape
Of the tawdry free
Dreaming dreaming in Honilee
For we are part of the never-ending,
Cascade of memory
Lending will to the snake
Shaping will and destiny
To the place of fear
As it watches us out of the cracks in things
That snake, that snake, that silver snake
Where does it go to hide?

Is it under the sun, under the earth?
Or in our minds
Or by the devils side
From yonder it came
That evil force
The swish of serpent
Twirling, hurling
Tumultuous tunnel rocketing
A surge of fishes
Sucked by its envy
Of majestic, furious streak
Bemused emotions dizzy, dizzy
For one last drag
To mock and damn us all
Where folk have evil souls
And the good are made to crawl
That snake that snake that silver snake
What will become of us?
The night on earth may be far too long
To haunt the slain
But it sneaks on us from the depths
And grows to immense size
To pounce and drag us down its hole
Too far to hear our cries
Ones who never escape
Their mingling in a bawdy room
Convincing others of their doom
As we frighten children witless
Until their mother drunk as fudge
Tucks the well heeled snake
Into a sprig of garlic
And is gone.

The apple was both fear and redemption. The "problem of pain," as the well-known Christian scholar, C.S. Lewis said, it is clear from both Scripture and universal experience that we are sinners by nature and thus will inevitably become sinners by choice as soon as we are able to do so. The sufferings of unsaved men are often recovered by the Holy Spirit to enable them to realize their need of salvation and to turn to Christ in repentance and faith. What a difficult job we have! In a fallen world, we try to do the right thing amidst a sea of wrongdoing we can barely keep afloat it seems - and then there was Jesus who made sense of it all. The sufferings of Christians should always be the means of developing a stronger dependence on God and a more Christ-like character, if they are properly "exercised thereby". *For we know that all things work together for good to them that love God, to them who are called according to His purpose* (Romans 8. 28).

An apple was passed to them. They took a bite and a youthful vigour they had long since lost was theirs. They stepped out of the ring and the change was their undoing. They lost the naivety and only had the blind ambition of youth. Malicious thoughts started to play on the body of waiting. Their minds were opening to a whole world of wisdom but they concentrated on its deceit and looking around they wanted. They just wanted. They wanted darkness. They had the seeds of the ages of the spiral tree and apple of youth. They wanted power. They wanted kinky group sex, drugs, filthy words, vats of chocolate, crates of coffee and beer; they wanted their reality with no consequence. The vampires glimpsed a raven flying overhead and looked up as they headed towards a group of buildings, chatting excitedly and very pleased with themselves, the majestic arrogance of youth restored. The god Loki transfixed me with a male power that engulfed him. The gods wanted him to steal back the apple. Spirit's Wonders Everlasting in the shape of the apple of youth did not conserve rather led to a state of youth's bliss.

"But I can do this thing" I insisted, "Yet the secret of youth will be given in return." Loki agreed as dawn came. The vampires locked the casket in a strong room and I opened a grate in the fireplace, room enough for the raven to enter via the chimney. The raven entered and upon finding the apples too heavy turned in his mind a hallowed spell to turn them to a single nut. Loki lifted it into the still morning air with his talons. The vampires, knowing that it was a plan by the gods gave chase, lifting their bat wings into the sky. The raven was growing old and he was slow. However as he reached the battlements of the gods they lit a huge fire. The raven passed through the flames but as the vampires approached they were singed and burnt and fell helpless to the ground dead. Psychosis in its beauty was the form of youth given and it happened between the candle and the flame. A wild imagination lost. There was no choice. I did not happen to it. It happened to me. Man in his original sin was reckless beyond efficiency. God therefore gave us free will from the gates of Eden, and to win our journey to the pods of eternity gave us the measurement of disorder and dismay, order and happiness. To act or be acted upon. Man wanted to act upon the world. Hence the plan to break the sound barrier. It collated mans' achievements as efficiency's constant brewed within him. But what had war taught us.

Realising something she could not realize - In a very small tunnel he sat. His hood was up; his nose was red with cold. Half-bugs crawled upon the crumpled newspaper he read and with fine determination; he brushed them into the air. They landed quickly, some running for their lives, some not. The Second World War was due anytime. He could hear police sirens on the streets and knew he was safe here. For a long time now, nothing had ever been complete. Even the cup he drank from was broken in two. He looked down to see if there had been any change in his lower limbs but they were still broken apart. Anxiously, he rubbed his rough whiskers looking upon nothing but devastation. Ever since that terrible day his village was bombed, he had been left with nothing but a broken box and a wish. For years, he had contemplated his destiny. Now he felt ready. The time had come for him to drag himself away, although in the back of his mind were thoughts that there would be nothing worse than to hear that whining again. Nevertheless, he had found some kind of inner strength and so heaved himself from this haven and shuffled cautiously on his way.

A trap had been set, but this had not fooled him. He could see it was also broken and not a threat. As he approached it, he felt a tension and to his horror the pain was immense - but he had not been touched. He cried tears that were some fifty years old, and as they fell, they left rusty lines on his cheeks continuing along to splash onto his filthy head. No one would find him here; no one would even hear his cries. He relaxed his broken body and wept for the sake of muse.

War took a sacrifice to convey to the world God's promise and raise the spirit in victory. To reverse evil upon good. This is where my perception of messiah came in. Does mental illness cause deformation by sin and reduce a man to sad conditions? It is rather because of it we resemble our Lord on the cross; it is the suffering image of God, but not a deformed image, inspired by the image of the Suffering Jesus without ability of assent required to sin. *What comes out of the mouth proceeds from the heart, and this defiles man* (Matthew 15:18). It is true that the objective disorder of sin and its consequences are manifest in the mentally ill patient; however, at the same time, there is in him the historical equilibrium of the only possible order, the order and equilibrium of the Redemption. Since the cross is the only way to the resurrection, the mentally ill person, has so to say a superior level, is worthier and reaches such a level of excellence because of the magnitude of his love and the suffering he endures. The mentally ill person is not a deformed image of God but, rather, a faithful image of Jesus. (Notes taken from a sermon by catholic bishop). The mentally ill person is making inroads to change a pattern of learnt behaviour, to soften broken souls where pockets of sinful residue had been left to gestate and grow and to join others in a bellowing cackle.

Mr Honity was the brains behind the plan, orchestrated by the military. He wanted me to find a seal which my uncle had lost and hence to win back heaven's failure during the war. *The reticent volcano keeps his never slumbering plan; confided are his projects pink to no precarious man. If nature will not tell the tale, Jehovah told to me, can human nature not survive without a listener be?* (E Dickinson) I saw references to it everywhere- from the gulf war news to films to poetry to Dickens. The only secret people keep is immortality. I saw it in the music of the Doors, Nirvana, Neil Young, and Danny Kaye. Finding a signed photo from Doris Day revealed that we were lovers and when she so majestically sang she was singing of the time barrier between us. I saw it in the science fiction, scientists, writers and artists of the 50's. I would read it from code in their work. Oh it was documented alright. Just in the subconsciousness of the establishment and counterculture of the time. You can interpret anything to mean what you meant it to mean but the military had to have their silence- listening to The Anti-Christ symphony by Peter Maxwell Davies while reading poetry on dead airmen called Michael by Yeats or Auden, I pieced together the story. If we were to know the truth, the elements of suspicion, fear, lies, deceit would no longer dull this dim land. Don't protect me by protecting me from the truth. We are all children in God's eyes.

Michael, you shall be renowned
When the demon you have drowned
A cathedral we will build
When the demon you have killed
When the demon is dead
You shall have a lovely clean bed

You shall be mine, all mine,
You shall have kisses like wine,
When the wine gets into your head
Mother will see that you're not misled;
A saint am I and a saint are you
It's perfectly, perfectly, perfectly true. (Auden)

     In my rapture I devised a code book in which I scrabbled down dream sequences and quotes from 50's science fiction and flight engineering books- to break Mr Honity's code which he had planted throughout history. My friend who was in a rock group found this book and looked at me in a knowing way. To this day I don't know if in his highly tuned rockstar mind he had a fait accompli with me all along and was in fact part of a clan of time travellers or whether he was saying- yeah its ok to be raving. Anyhow he used to say that inspiration for his songs simply fell in his lap from the sky. This is how I found it. Years of pie in the sky.

     I understood that my uncle, Michael Warrick was the pilot who would complete the mission from Waterbeach airfield in Cambridgeshire. A jet plane "The Mongoose" was designed by the aircraft company De Havilland in Hatfield to rival the rocket experiments in America. Icarus flew too near the sun, which isn't a safe or friendly place for wax to be. The error lay in the lack of respect for the nature of his materials. His mistake wasn't in trying to fly. That comes with the territory of being human. It was understood that the boundary layer would not allow traditional structures to withstand the shock waves associated with the speed of sound. The early jets experienced the forces involved, often catastrophically. Those such as the meteor were built as platforms for the jet engine, not necessarily for the velocities involved. If wonderful works were easily translated by human reason they would not be wonderful. A flight of ideas? Just running away from the truth faster than my legs could carry me. No wonder losing weight was on the agenda, my anxious thoughts expended as much energy as running a marathon with one of those all-in-one fun costumes on, guaranteed to feel suffocating and cause overheating and going through fits and starts - not dissimilar to the exhausting battle experienced daily on psychiatric medication.

On a hill in Plymouth, I gathered speed one cold autumn evening. I knew my intention. The coloured leaves were lifting in the strong wind and for a time so did I. Fully conscious I experienced flight in just the same time as you can perhaps lose your keys and not be aware of what you did to lose them. Flying became like a broken arrow to me which showed whenever the memory laps over the drag of the aircraft and countenance became the heart of man grafting a slow heading from the merriment and contentment of equity with nature to strike hammer purposed through the moving air like a propeller blade. Desperation and instinct drained a long sigh, holding their purpose flighty under the pale countenance and reflection, communing with the rush of the engines, the wings cutting through the pressure of nature's invisible art in the sky beyond them. From energies to the images so came the imaginative, and the desired so that the forces within the cosmos, my achievements, qualities, belief, commitment and opinions flew in space and time like a small breeze lifted heavenly toward the horizon. Those creaking sails keep sounding her fayre, the gull's whip is bare, and I breathe in purity. We moved in a butterfly's gasp; the wings that roamed full of the giggling naive compassion of a vision sealed in innocence. I swooped and still we swept upwards. She would seek. She thought. She would find. She thought under the pale countenance and reflection, desperation and instinct like Venus first held confidence with Vulcan.

Nevertheless, it was enough for me to feel exhilarated. Afterwards, I returned to my flat to eat yet another plate of pasta and practice some scales. Of course, I wanted to tell of my groundless adventure but no one would believe me. So, I assumed that the sound barrier was a code in the twentieth century for a much larger function. Understanding the forces of nature which were all held together by spectral diversity in the ratio of phi. A shock wave forms on the aircraft when it reaches supersonic speeds. From the front of the plane, the shock wave appears as a circle, but from the back and sides, it looks like very sharp spikes coming off of the plane. It is a rare and spectacular sight, only visible in humid weather. This, I thought, was God's code supplanted throughout nature to bind together creation. No one knew whether we could survive a sonic boom or that it would simply shake our atoms apart.

In the Grip of the Rippling Thrice
Bright and twinkling the stars unfold
Futures bright and manifold
All yesterday's tomorrow's creation
Is nature's code
Of spectral diversity
Swears to our eyes from phi
A ratio contained in the double helix
From bodies whose ashes cover 2 feet of the globe
To yield us bread.
Reclaim the power of nature
Retrieve the night with the power of electrons
At the speed of light

In natures loftiness
See the precise arrangement of petals
Animate past forests with a lump of coal
Receive grand regions of the soul with perception
Moulded by their relationship with phi.
The majestic geometry of flowers
The movement of bird on wing
The double helix of genes
All these passions find a heart
Like a shell's spiral delivering sound
From the sea's holy tide
Affected by the moon's round
Dappled bounty at our feet
Phi the element of truth
Where nature and God meet
Contained in dimensions
Contained in our blueprint
Yet in the language of a computer
Bright and twinkling the stars unfold
Futures bright and manifold
What if heaven should fail?
All yesterday's tomorrow's creation
Is nature's code
Of spectral diversity.

Chapter 2 Dandelion Time

The subject, the Illusion, the illumination: In a multitude of bleary eyes. So tantalize my bravest fear but grant me peace for one last chance among a glance so strong, so loud. Let me be proud. To stand aside this poverty- perhaps their peek may freely shriek. When they do dream (and they will dream) of gaiety and carefree days, so full of wistful, wildly twist; no speech will sound yet silence brings no alibi.

People will try to help but it is really one's own choices that count towards rehabilitation. There is no alibi between the candle and the flame. Many mental health issues are now being seen through the eyes of the carer and sufferer. *God shall wipe away all tears from their eyes; and there shall be no more death, neither sorrow, nor crying, neither shall there be any more pain* (Revelation 21. 4). No more than Plato's lullaby can rock a mortal safely by, the price of madness, the space between illusion and illumination, is often to lose the subject.

Tabatha tindermouse lived in a dark damp cellar that exhibited gravel floors, damp doorways and skeletons of her ancestors. She stroked a rib cage in fond memory and as she looked up, her eyes par-blind from the dust and rottings from the walls refused to shame her. A rusted built in bread oven some seven-foot deep cried out for restoration and so did she. Her squeak was met at the top of the cellar entrance by a laugh-if-you-care laddermouse. He approached her situation with disdain bringing with him the arm of a bat and a tadpole's tail. 'Make it happen' he conjected. The blue of his cataract eyes shined back at her through the moonlight glare that Tumnus the puss-cat had bottled. Tumnus always said that it was a fine year for moon juicing. The year before the London festival of

Olympics. He had been in training every day for six hours at least and was to be the favourite among the hurdlers. Tabatha gathered her thoughts to realize how many years she had spent in anti-training for the event. Yet something she knew was not so it seemed with laugh-if-you-care. His determination equalled his struggle plus a generous helping of guilt. Yet out of his dry, uncouth mouth came the sweetest song.

I cannot tell her it's not my place to say but yes
I'll be there to pick up the pieces, I'm afraid
Does she try, or does she not, well I don't care for image
But she sits and she waits by the ivory gates and shudders

Please don't cry little girl
I know you're to blame,
You know you're to blame
But what's the use now
We can't look back, can't go back to
Yesterday's market place

Things for sale, new and old, in a rush
I wipe your tears away
I tried to tell you but
I was afraid

In a ring all shouting
Their wares, all-staring
Faces all laughter but
Can't they see what I see?
Why can't they see what I see?
The terror in their eyes
The terror they're feeding us
Terror they're bleeding us

I know you're to blame,

You know you're to blame
But what's the use now
We can't look back, can't go back to
Yesterday's market place

So where do you start telling
Someone you love them
When they show cracks beyond repair

And I know she's not fine
And she tries hard to please me
But I can tell and the truth is
That I'm suffering more for her suffering
Than that little girl

Please don't cry little girl
Please don't cry
Please don't cry little girl

Off you go, go back
Go on go, go and play
Little girl so young, off you go, go back
Go back to yesterday's
Marketplace

Then laugh-if-you-care laddermouse walked quietly
away from the broken mirror he had been looking
through and away, up the cellar stairs he crept clutching
his bat arm and tadpole tail, not to be seen for longer
than a while.

A tattered and scared path appeared in front of
our dreams leading to a majestic mantle in the sky,
circling an apogee of sharing beneath the stars of lost
reminders. I suppose that if friends go off on tangents,
mine more heavily than anyone else's, then relations
are sure to drift. I have the distinct memory of others
climbing the greasy pole with such consummate pace

that I remember the unpredictability I may have shown and hence the guilt mixed with resentment and inadequacy. Maybe just the concept of justice was misled somewhere in the affray. Loyalty like a pilot never really dies. It just mutates. *Memory of sunflower, bees and bluebottle's sunshine till the dawn he writes with a gabbling pen tardily. No onions for a while, doors open, shadows fall. Embers of an Elizabethan hunt they glow bright in meadows pasture. She wore her pigtails well- historic figments as pigments the glitter of her golden age dreams of the honeysuckle sand in bloom. Sparkling suns for everyone. In a beachscape land. Who are you? What do you want? Still haunted by the whisper; what's the point of it all? Alas some questions fail answers and just as well cos the path is rosy. Every path has its rose. And every rose its thorn. Between the candle and the flame all was grey until at this age of understanding, she stepped off the path.* (O. Dachinger)

Find a way or make a way was carved on the seacave's tidal mark. It was as though gryphons were waiting to carry us from this reality into a different one, for there was the pod, and it was familiar to me as I waited many a time, waited to follow Angel'rain through the portal which shone like a glassy sea. Sometimes I would wait in this pod of eternity and like the double helix in genes some thoughts come from within. So it was when I was there, in the pod, killing time. The pod was the green rusting colour of metal. Riveted panels like the innards of a submarine. Faith was all that remained there. Like the gaze of a lighthouse (the medical profession she had once said) I looked into her eyes to judge in a place such as this.

"Please try to avoid me
You will reel in dreadful pain
Without even knowing dreadful pain
I try to warn you

My gaze, my gaze
Is too splendid

I can witness you diminish
Hear you claw and fight
Against a thunderous salt slap
I try to warn you
My gaze, my gaze
Has chewed you up

Across the limpet cloth you blurt
Stabbing an anchor aimlessly
A net so full of caught hope
I try to warn you
My gaze, my gaze
Has tort you"

We muse on the glassy sea-like portal, which passed
from the night to day. A spillage of cyclamen pushes its
way across, scattered the broken buds, candle still to
the fall. I tasted not the sweet honey for fear of its
deathly sting.

I never hear the word escape
Without a quicker blood
A sudden expectation
A flying attitude

I never hear of prisons broad
By soldiers battered down
But I tug childish at my bars
Only to fail again (Emily Dickinson)

Above the pod was a windsock blowing in the
wind of our discontent: the resentment, disbelief,
crowded with the transgressions of life. The windsock
shows faith's direction of the open future and present,
one of hope and gladness. Led by both fairy chance of

sayings and choice we were battered by authority to be content to kill time- but by killing time we injure eternity. Black stars cast their shadows, radiant though they seem. The ebony star needs not the brightness of day to extinquish. It does not care for the sun's power. Through the sky, psychotic dreams pretend, threatening an elegant gaze weakening an admirers bond. I fall next to a broken dream, no longer to share the moon with the woman in white. The sea, a puddle riddled with effortless rain, refuses its reflection. She reflected on the afterglow. Angel'rain whispered "Dear moon where do you tread, face me here this night, tell me your will oh salient friend, my tears are for you". For the glance down the moonlit cove when all is said and spelt there is but one thing that remains in the windsock. Faith of what I don't see and hope in what I do.

So in Tabatha's winter store went all things fearsome and dreadful. Out she ventured to gather nuts in May and butts by day – rights by lords and wrongs in hoards in preparation for her self evaluation (that would hopefully be so insignificant at that point that all would be well). A barmy way of going on, and one truly sticky situation to eradicate oneself from. Heady days. When that dark day struck, there was no question. Her mouth could not speak save a throaty writhsome shriek as the moths gathered strength to cascade and pursue as busy and uncouth as a large umbrella opening and shutting in your face. The stirring air was enough to startle the small rodents from their occupations. Dizzily she span until mad eyed and panting, she leapt to a corner with a blanket for safe keeping and just stayed put. Was it worth living this to juicily document a right scene? Maybe? Maybe not. Perhaps to keep to the long enduring 'how d'you do's' and 'spiffing fancy's' might be a step or rather quite a few in a certain direction.

In our soul's windsock
The majestic soul arises
From wind direction
And accepts its moments creep
To a risen soul as proof
Leaps over understanding
The love of trying keeps
Full circle with faith
To transfigure our souls
And take over destiny
From faith's dimension shifting
That our reality assumes
The windsock
Measures the human condition
And allows us to decide
And show ourselves
In expression and beauty
Stalking the crucibles rim
For balance to restore

"Decisions are often taken through the lens of medication." Angel'rain said "- until entropy's tendency to disorder finally curtails our choices. Now these shadows I recognize as we sit debating judgements breath, a turmoiled procession scatters, splinters but does not explain the pain of just dying slowly. 'Tis the ultimate endgame of entropy's answer of order descending to disorder. Order is created by medication but at what cost? Is the striving for arts and sciences to be part of medical knowledge? Something loses its validity. Not simply shock but hiding pain. But medical practice does not involve punishment. Like a dog that won't walk nicely next to me so I wore the psychiatric nose harness. The problem of mine was that I was endangered by my inability to see the wood from the trees and see what conditions were in other people's minds and to see where I fitted in with all the personal jealousies and resentments that go along with relations coupled with drug use. To give me drugs and lock me into power trips with sadistic intentions was not very clever. Strive against the dimming of the day if ever you are in that position. Read poetry, read minds but certainly don't read your medical notes! I had a dead uncle and all he ever wrote was night follows the day and day follows the night. He died in 1953 in a plane, a silver experimental plane trying to break the sound barrier:

How wonderful is Death,
Death and his brother Sleep!
One pale as yonder wan and horned moon,
With lips of lurid blue,
The other glowing like... the space
Between the candle and the flame...
Yet both so passing strange and wonderful!
In light of some sublimest mind, decay?
Nor putrefaction's breath
Hark! Whence that rushing sound?
'Tis like a wondrous strain that sweeps
Around a lonely ruin
When west winds sigh and evening waves respond
In whispers from the shore:
'Tis wilder than the unmeasured notes
Which from the unseen lyres of dells and groves
The genii of the breezes sweep.
Floating on waves of music and of light,
The chariot of the Daemon of the World (Shelley)

Yet does that make him any less real than those standing aloof by your side? Telling the story like clockwork? The desolate clocks stand in rows; solitary, silent; in penitence for their awakening- yet Michael and I would lie there for each other in times of indecision like the breaking of the time barrier. They just announce the time like it was something new. We knew time. Life as we know it is now. A moment in time. A brief moment in the universe, following the language of curiosity, following an arrow of time governed by the second law of thermodynamics and its principle of entropy increase. This says that order will most likely descend to chaos and is the explanation of time, as we perceive it:

If time could breathe
It would never sustain such elements as these

Motionless knot
And powerless neither
Maker of war
Dictator of tongues

If I could turn suns
And multiply trees
And multiply people
Would I prove the constant?
Would I turn a suffering into years of despair?

Yet time advanced to let me breathe. To show me it was possible to overcome all of this. I look forward to when I reach that time again in real time. A catalyst is necessary sometimes when all else fails. So strong a freedom was reached that absolutely everything was settled, everything was ok and everything was going to be manageable. I stood in a Loughton car park outside the mental health centre. This was when time truly slowed to reveal an accepted euphoria. The ease I felt similar to floating on water under a clear blue sky – unspoiled. A good person showed me this place. A car park, full of cars and an agitated traffic warden itching to do his job. Not the nicest of places you may think. But here it was. Heaven. I just wait for that time again. I believe it will be reached but I would love to say it would last longer than the afternoon it lasted there. It was then that the balloon returned to the ground.

The revelation first occurred to me in a shop "On seeing the time barrier for the first time, the eye is completely dazzled by the rich variety of illumination; and it is not until this partial bewilderment has subsided, that we are in a condition to appreciate as it deserves its real magnificence and the harmonious beauty of effect produced by the artistical arrangement of the glowing and varied hues which blaze along its grand and simple lines... Triumph of man exploding the myth of Law... It affords a true test of the point of development at which the whole of mankind has arrived in this great task, and a new starting point from which we are able to direct our further exertions...

Time protruding from a crack was like the fingers of the empire, or so it seemed, which clasped the dreams of madmen among the wares, which were on display here. The antique clocks had captivated the factors of production- labour, markets and raw materials. They were the ramifications of this industrial revolution. We were tellers of the regimented industrial age, an age of egalitarian idealists who had given up the harmony of agriculture and selected regimentalism at the hands of the clock. The movement of time did not conserve rather led to a state when a process was repetitive beyond efficiency. The temporal nature of life and the entropy that seems to point towards the relationship between time and disorder is not God's plan? What if a moment of time, death, could lead to life? Religion has a name for it, namely, resurrection. Ok, so many psychotics believe they are messiah. But the Christian belief is that we are all a part of Jesus and hence we all have eternal life: spirit's wonders everlasting:

Entropy did not conserve
Rather led to a state
When a process beguiles
Footfalls on a desolate shore
Man in his original sin
Reckless beyond efficiency
Spirit's wonders everlasting
Bright and twinkling to Jesus
But the journey of our souls
Energy's answer to win
Our journey to the pods of eternity
A measurement of disorder
Efficiency's constant to collate
Upon a windswept apogee
Of Earth's great livery
And spread our meteor plumes
Rising by God's secret sap
The majestic soul arises
From the deep cavernous sleep
And accepts its moments creep
To a risen soul as proof
Leaps over understanding
The love of trying keeps
Full circle with faith
To transfigure our souls
From faith's dimension shifting
That our reality assumes
Entropy's shadow
Measures the human condition
For the Lord's love is like moonlight
Its fronds a happy home beneath
Joy by which angels do fly
Gladness seeping from their wings
Stalking the crucible's rim
For balance to restore
Triumph of man exploding
The myth of God and Law
The changes of entropy

Are but the spirit's
Gentler equation imploring you
To inspire and regulate time so far
Entropy of spirit enchanting
For science to encounter
True reversibility
Like a carpet of riverbed moss
To find balance where there is chaos
Entropy's answer is shown
Tends to collective purpose.

Measurement of disorder began by trains, timetables and industry to collate upon a windswept apogee of earths great livery, were the spreading of clock hands by God's secret sap. "When the footfalls were one it was when I was carrying you" chimed the dandelion clock. It was really something to hear your voice and thoughts over all these years. What shall I say to you? Here I sit, in a strange room, in a strange land, and my life lies behind me. It is close upon midnight, and very dark. I can see nothing out of window. The air is hot and heavy, the moths flutter round my candle; I cannot save them all. I am trying to write you a letter— do you understand? The clock ticks incessantly. Time must have a stop. Oh, but I have no thoughts, only visions! The more I felt alienated by the city types the more I listened to music and to the wooden echoes of the trees and such and the only thing I can say is that I tried to take footfalls with the grace they deserved and saw the best in people. I suppose you get the chances to tie together lifestrings in art and science and it's hard not to see the flaws in yourself but these are the very things that we have taken delight in. Cawing against the dimming of the day. I had a dead uncle once and the only thing he ever wrote was the day follows the night and night follows the day. He that followeth me shall not walk in darkness, saith the Lord. His reality assumed a shift. Entropy's shadow measured the human condition for a dandelion's love is like moonlight; its fronds joy by which angels fly.

"I must buy that clock," I said. At that very moment on the stall next to me psychosis's hand reached out to buy... the other Dandelion clock. A tattered and scared road appeared in front of our dreams leading to a mantle in the sky, circling an apogee of sharing beneath the stars of lost reminders. Shall heaven fail me? Wrapping these clocks up in all his charms- prowess seemed a long way away as we passed glances for a second but it seemed like an age we connected, a rare connection that only happens once or twice in a lifetime- a real one off. It was said that each tomorrow was to be a tender disappointment but also a wonderful experience. I handed over my currency and left with the packages under my arm. Ambiguity stalked London's rim as he walked the dirty streets home for balance to restore.

"Why would I like spiralling around and around and around?" said psychosis. Normality felt like a circling wheel with fuzzy boundaries- a mere spectator circling through an ordinary day. We had responded to the motivation of dreams to avoid the atrocities of the socio-economic pressures that acted on London's migrants. Sections of the city had developed into places of finance of banks insurance and exchanges, older companies, docks, retail establishments and residential areas. Residential areas were at first respectable then grew into shock slums as many pioneers found the life too difficult and whose physical and mental well being suffered or gambled or drunk their lives away. The piggeries and linen row were the urban slums of the city situated within breathing space of the rich. Spillage from industry and inroads of mental health with its long hours, gambling and lowliness breathed its stench into the vanities of the rich businessmen and landowners of the London scene. Hurrying clerks leaving the city on the new Metropolitan and district tube lines to pigeon-haunted classic towers saw the fleet and Cheapside slums as only a fearful step away. A clock chime away. Yet this was a long time ago, and I remembered it fondly as our first shared experience of London.

The daily pattern and rhythm of his life led him to be disappointed. The wild mood-swings would chill his loneliness to the bone. But psychosis coveted time. That we ought to be thankful remembering the clock gives the grace, it makes the choice of collective purpose and perhaps the temptation is to just play safe. To squander choice and just deal in damage limitation. Atlas held the world aloft to enchant like a carpet of riverbed moss- to find balance where there is chaos. So it was that the connection with Mr Honity kept precious pearls building inside of them, precious pearls which mixed with formative experiences and illuminated that part of them which is not still as a photograph, still as the vixen in whose screams I try to see some love, something more than lustily impregnated desire. Yet the pendulum swings order in chaos for they had always absorbed new experiences like the dial face, full of flashes of light and statement, substance and creativity and our loneliness had always moved in ever decreasing circles.

To co-operate with the clocks' grace is to make ourselves vulnerable, to open the way to a portal between minds is to open ourselves to the possibilities within us. The clocks ticked as one looked upon their sweeping repetitiveness of time as lives impressed by one another's. I am more impressionable when my cement is wet. I move from high entropy (wet clay) to low entropy (sculpture). The connection of time is to receive each other's call to do his/her will. It was a revelation of a calling in life. One just had to become entranced by the slowing down of each moment and if you listen there was a voice calling you to action.

Sometimes subtle it can be a definite push and so it was I found the inner strength to break the bonds with the only places they had ever known, concrete grey.

How do we make decisions? Moving from high entropy (chaos) to low entropy (rationality) is the normal thought pattern but the second law of thermodynamics comes into play during psychosis, as it is far more likely that chaos gets out of control. Psychosis is a way of getting control and many with a sickening reliance on sanity revert to the wrong decisions anyway. Deciding in and out of reality is a common feature in everyone's lives. There is always that inner voice separate from the outside world so concrete grey which seems to overcome the principle of entropy increase. My way of dealing with the outside world was to use my uncle's inner voice.

The trouble with the outside world is that it cannot be kept at bay appreciating again that people are wonderful creatures, full of character, culture, breeding and imagination- so I became obsessed with this pilot who seemed to have life sorted out to resolve our doubts in such a way as to allay our fears. No rawness faded in the rapture of the dead pilot and his example. I slink off into bed mildly curious for I do not lay this candle to rest like his ghost, which moved through me some nights. The green shroud it wore will never let fade. It shrouds the mechanism by which all my future loves have been gauged. That carefree, poignant, mischievous, deliquesce tick-tock- innocent motivation between the quandaries- virtue and trust are distracted by... tick-tock... power and sex- mutually transferable but in between there is calm, still like the mist that surround the two clocks who have discovered... fleetingly... tick-tock... synchronicity.

Synchronicity creates
A mirror
Innocent arches and sparkles extreme
That psychosis shatters
On the midpoint of now
And deposits on the time line
Past and present and future
Full of many cherished moments
Exploding in pinnacles of light
Like the splendour of firelight
As the day growing dim
Harks us a magnificent deed
And plays us a hymn
With shadow like grace
And eyes aglow
Concealing ceaseless reflection
With impetus, vigour and low
The mirror's wonders everlasting
Bright and twinkling to Jesus
Are but the journey of our souls.
Upon a windswept apogee
Of earths great livery
And spread our meteor plumes
Rising by God's secret sap
The majestic reflection arises
From the deep cavernous sleep
And accepts its moments creep
To a risen soul as proof
Leaps over understanding
The love of trying keeps
Full circle with faith
To transfigure our souls
From faith's dimension shifting
That our reality assumes
Mirror's barrier in heaven's shadow
Yonder broken
Communication of intimacy
Our souls alight

That if heaven should fail
The mirror like a spindle
True grace of extraordinary
Spinning a tapestry of light
Portraying the rapture you kindle
Will be our reflection of God

Chapter 3 Eternity Beach

Eternity beach is real we are just artificial seeds sewn to conquer its thoughts and aspirations. We approach the pods in the cavern like they were washed up coconuts on the shoreline. The most important thing is to remember that we all, whoever we are, have good intentions- everyone instinctively recognizes that "good" is a higher order of truth than "bad". *For we know that all things work together for good to them that love God, to them who are called according to His purpose* (Romans 8.28). From the beginning to the end this was the plan. In your own lifetime one has chances but is death the end of time?

Grant for a moment, that there is a realm beyond our senses. Let us agree that from his earliest beginnings man has created gods in whom just the deadly and menacing and destructive and terrifying elements in life were contained- its violence, its fury, its impersonal bewilderment- all tied together into one thick knot of malevolence: something alien to us, if you wish, but something which let us admit that we were aware of it, endured it, even acknowledged it for the sake of a sure, mysterious relationship and inclusion in it; for WE WERE THIS TOO; only we didn't know what to do with this side of our experience; it was too large, too dangerous, too many sided, it grew above and beyond us, into an excess of meaning; we found it impossible (what with the demands of a life adapted to habit and achievement) to deal with these unwieldy and ungraspable forces; and so we agreed to place them outside US- but since they were an overflow of our own being, its most powerful element, indeed were TOO powerful, were huge, violent, incomprehensible, often monstrous-: how could they not, concentrated in one place exert an influence and ascendancy over us? And, remember from the outside now, couldn't the history of

God be treated as an almost never-explored area of the human soul, one that has always been postponed, saved, and finally neglected...?

And then, you see, the same thing happened with death. Experienced, yet not to be fully experienced by us in its reality, continually overshadowing us yet never truly acknowledged, forever violating and surpassing the meaning of life- it too was banished and expelled, so that it might not constantly interrupt us in the search for this meaning. Death, which is probably so close to us that the distance between it and the life centre inside us cannot be measured, now becomes something external, held further away from us every day, a presence that lured somewhere in the void, ready to pounce upon this person or that in its evil choice. More and more the suspicion grew up against death that it was the contradiction, the adversary, the invisible opposite in the air, the force that makes all our joys wither, the perilous glass of our happiness, out of which we may be spilled at any moment....

All this might still have made a kind of sense if we had been able to keep God and death at a distance, as mere ideas in the realm of the mind: but nature knew nothing of this banishment that we had somehow accomplished- when a tree blossoms, death as well as life blossoms in it, and the field is full of death, which from its reclining face sends forth a rich expression of life, and the animals more patiently from one to the other- and everywhere around us, death is at home, and it watches us out of the cracks in things, and a rusty nail that sticks out of a plant somewhere, does nothing day and night except rejoice over death. (Patrick Duff)

Deep within the heart of the whispering cavern, we approached a velvet lupine pod. I stroked its side and raising its hairs, it sighed in appreciation. How soft and warm it felt. It gradually opened a glassy portal and showing no resistance we jumped through. Inside the pod is quite different, like the tardis. Its walls are polished green and smell so fresh, so new. There were two impressions left on one side, one of you and one of I as we sit perfectly in these moulds, we sing folk tunes. The pod beats calmly in approval. I dream of salvation as a revelation to stay on the path to heaven so that the end is not watching my own grave like a Dickensian saga. Being pretty and clever never got anyone anywhere, and our aspirations are realised through fantasy. Backstage the theme progressed as a kind of Hitchcockian whodunit. The feeling was that I had to save the world and all I had was a stick. The feeling of my old school pervaded the atmosphere and I frantically ran from auditorium to corridors and back rooms searching.

Then to a castle by a river, the set of the play. Someone had just won a sailing race and I had to enter to be runner up. Honour was at stake. I got a wooden ironing board I presume. I got a clasp and string from a greenhouse and friends would be making me a sail. Then I was sitting on the shore and a man, a kindly man gave me a banana stick. After I had constructed the boat, by putting the stick in a knot in the wood and fixing the clasp to the top of the pole, I just went around banging people over the head depending on whether they had lived good lives or not. To sail the race there was a feeling akin to first seeing mountains on a train journey into Swansea. This feeling of eternity or coming home is displayed in a portal in the pod and are of the same construction as the awe in which I first saw them rising above the train track in Wales. I look above and behold the image of a beautiful being glowing on the shiny surface. The eyes so stunning, of the deepest blue, portray innocence that only God would have permission to paint, lashes thick and so neatly ordered that each curls correctly (and I use this term because no other arrangement could be considered as perfect as this). However viewed as a glossy spectacle they look somehow glazed, somehow sad.

The whole is inconceivable to the imagination, the hair forming the most beautiful golden haze. The lips perfectly formed, the outline delicately suggested. They just long to be kissed. But because of the nature of its canvas this porcelain portrait is of a rather sickly countenance. The apple cheeks blushed in defence of nature's flourishing hue. The vision remained only long enough for it to be absorbed by the mind and upper casing of the pod. It faded naturally until it was nothing but a memory. It was the alien who had created this portal. To revive such an episode I knew was impossible, as when viewing such splendour, not only did the experience yield visual beauty- imagine the music that rushed at the sight- imagine the emotions. Only then would one begin to understand the power this helpless cherub encompassed, the power to transform peace into ecstatic chaos. The power to tune the senses to such acuteness that the eyes see like the deaf and the ears hear like the blind. But even it was unaware, for opposite us on the far side of the pod, there was another glassy portal. It beckoned our arousal and shone of an alien beach, familiar, as it was strange. Echo beach far away in time. We jumped through.

When I jumped through the portal it was an analogy of anticipation and fantasy coupled with the expectation that ignorance is bliss. I would turn the cross earring in the rock by the side and stop any other undesirable from following me. There were friends and sun and sea in echo beach but a strange alien sea from many millennia ago. It was red, red as a sea of poppies and there were two moons. Savour the aroma of bliss, not a drug to be seen except the memory of death ringing out a chilling red as the vibrant melody line piercing the darkest edges of my soul while the thin harmonics, thin as a chain of snowflakes, frozen in wonder as through a moths wing, powdery as opiate, illustrate the irony of a poppy. The blasphemous sea rocked to and fro in its ladle sustaining the freshness of the air. Was this ocean's juice derived from sadness or joy of another sort? We wondered as it continued to choke all who glanced but feed those who dared. *A blood-red papery crepe doily so demure and handsome until all that is left is the bombastic seed-core, black as night to be harvested by the oncoming ant brigade and they march on just like those soldiers of old, searching for heroics, finding the warping, the epiphany of truth…perhaps.* (O. Dachinger)

To and fro, its tumultuous tide regained strength and the skinless fruits shed their pips and marched to the profane polyphony of a thousand seagulls in search of revolution. A ship appeared on the horizon but turned to a wreck from an old Turner painting as it approached. Spores of alcoholic themes drowned the mast producing further spores until the rich punch became a reeking puree of incestuous delight for the consumption of those desperate enough to sin at the feet of the sinner. How their ears and tongues burned as they revelled in their own heaving hope of heaven. Sailors had been here before and it was a place of expectations and fruitfulness but tinged with desperation of the sea's red glow. A world that could be home if only we would share our light of balanced moments. The balanced moment is the space between the candle and the flame like a small increment in time or a lifetime in the scale of the universe. Described in Mathematics as a small change in one over a small change in another it is the time lapse between the sound and the hearing- the space between moments. A human life to God perhaps? The portal showed us what the alien's saw.

Always there would be Angel'rain and she would tell me of the vast histories of the planet and before time began, memories of an alien race who carved out existence in the sea in front of us and had left residues of memory in each and every creature. They built the portals and pod of eternity but whom had long since left to travel space. They were brain like creations that had left their mark on the world by creating animal brains from their image. Their blueprint for humans was shown to us previously as we entered the pod. But this was all in memory. Like fragments of memories from dreams, reality draws you back like the tide or dawn. The warm earth breathed and could be heard throughout the heavens-   they had been waiting for this time. Angel'rain and I stood, expectantly, on the alien beach shore. The silent rain dropped calmly cooling its surface and soothing its cracks and a shoot was born, perfect, and steady, it stretched and saw for the first time amid the warm earth sighed. Peering across the land at distant plains, it shone and grew - the symbol of new life. My master had arrived and would ascend to greater heights and I continued to patter such a delicate bud. The butterflies rejoiced as they danced around him and ascending at his pace, fluttered on his pale green skin. They kissed each other and tasted the sweet nectar on his side and each kiss produced a butterfly blossom. They were in paradise and so was he. Nothing could be better than this, the sun shone, the breeze from the multitude of wings was light and I continued to protect you above and underground. I penetrated the warm earth in search of your roots so that you may grow stronger and faster. Like a magnet I was drawn to your soul in search of existence and finally resumed physical state - with you. We were both stronger now and soared for the sake of each other passionately piercing the clouds of betrayal and scattering new seeds for the warm earth to contemplate. We rose passed all of this and more and more we grew, until you brought me to the steps of eternal light. This was as they had expected and all was well. There was a gentle stirring from the east side of the voids albumen and an inquisitive shudder was felt among. The sound and vibrations were dampened though and did not wake the floating fruits from their pleasurable sleep.

This is the beach and I welcome you here on behalf of those who have already realized their wishes and desires. Everyone is here, look up and you will see stars, look closer and around, now fly up and stroke them softly and, you see, these stars are not. They are forms waiting to be discovered - but only they may discover themselves and until then they offer the beach what light they can from the far distance. We all have subconsciously resided here, even before we were born but once arrived, we feel an ease that is too beautiful to imagine but can only be felt. A serene and pure energy that holds all beachcombers in exquisite delight. How come you ventured through Narnia to this cove? Had you tried to find me there? I only reside there on occasion, when I think too often for my soul to stand. It is cold there but never too cold. I like the fresh mist and well being that follows and the rose petals that brush my skin and tickle my temples. The petals transform as my soul is replenished into pieces of pink fluffy blossoms. They taste sweet and provide energy and from there I can continue to diddle in the depths of the firmament.

Time is of no essence now; you dwell forever among and within each of us, extracting eternal love and light when you wish. Michael who escaped the flood of poppies, approached death with intrigue, I am not depressed, just intrigued. He had been content to value his life without fear, fear in all of their eyes and ours of isolation. A feeling of constancy, a plane wed in my head ushering in the cure. Friends and partygoers, animalistic, gave money and paid for a prostitute. Jesus as a sphere, and we as tide's followers sang a-ring-a-ring-a-roses. The beach was like a final place, a pre-primary point for eternity and love. And now for the subject of love. I am no expert (I don't think anyone can claim to be) but I know I have felt pain many times and each prick singes a nerve that becomes dead forever. You know master, I detest the practicality that life has to offer, and I simply detest it. I detest standing next to the one that drained me of everything at the bus stop every morning. I detest being cheated, fucked and pitied. I do not wish to be old but there is nothing we can do. There is nothing we can do about the formalities of life. Try and oppose it and nothing but a pathetic statement is made, still we are part of its tomb. Our bodies grow no younger, our thoughts grow no younger. And all I want to do is hide. I do admire the turning point.

I have been the taker
Not of my own accord
Whose Life had been rattled
'Til the shaker dispersed

And now on the other side
I stand almost tall
Away from the cruel mirror
I glared at for too many years

I have a turning point to thank
And for being, I thank you
You have made me whole.

For showing me the way
I thank those who love me
Especially god and myself

No lies, no hiding, no shame
No one to blame

Just circumstance of a twisted society
The human is a curious phenomenon

No more fear of us
Only intrigue, excitement and understanding

Now for the future in the pale moonlight for it glowed resplendent on the seashore. The brain like creatures implored us to join them with swishing tentacles. But they had long since returned to space whence they had come. The warm earth breathed and could be heard throughout the heavens- they had been waiting for this time. The sand was cold and wet and it began to grow, so far it grew that I could no longer see the stars and then I realized that we had sunk to its very soul. Should we have been aware of such a discovery before? How much longer can we keep on going? How much longer can it last? After all, this soul is useless to everybody but the sand and then, after years of cultivation and manipulation; some new wave could come along and destroy its very history, its starting point, and its finishing point. And yes we chuckle; they would destroy its finishing point. I turn to you and hold out my hand, you take hold of my fingers and we utter words of our hearts into the sand:

Comfort me.
Of all the times that seconds have ticked so monotously, this is the time I need not hear them.
Comfort me.
And I shall offer comfort in return.
In shallow waters we may wade pitifully to where -
The shiny creature lays,
Resting on the dunes of weirdom, waiting.
Comfort me.
And through all eternity we shall fall and rise and fall together.
For this is all we can do now - we are capable to only

imagine
What is beheld in the sand's most active paths
For we have been destined to reach the soul.

Chapter 4 Name, Rank and Number

From the case spills his uniform like a blackened bull. Stars glittering here and there, distantly in his warm hands he smelt Mars, of iron and the planet Venus, a green ivy smell and the planet mercury, a scent of sulphur and fire and he could smell the milky moon, milky white and glowing with a light of its own. If dawn could gait a thousand stars, my eyes would envelope a more tender heart, but lack of knowing what God knows best, shines through our souls and keeps us blest. I thought I heard a trumpet call? Sedentary tones, yet full of warmth, no piercing shriek hit still our minds; just "Danny boy" came rolling home. I waited with bated breath as the walls turned from purples to mist and through this mist my mother and I heard his footsteps on the street below. To stare at the oak, for time it tells t'ward a breath not gasp, expel our branches intertwine and grow, shoots bud and flowers sweet scent flow. First disembarking the MG, then turning the street corner then footsteps up the path. I know I can be what you want. You may not challenge what you want, your sweet embrace, a dance, a sip to your sweet nature gently I trip. Both would lie awake for hours to hear this through eyes to tell the tale, orange passion, haze surreal, fizzes to a surface-ray effervescence, true brilliance of souls, our sweet embrace to find out why the tangent breaks a circle. Gently now, come rest your place, gently now come rest your case. You are my giant among the stars and they shine on you, illumine Mars.

I found in the pendulum swaying heights of life a movement of heart stopping, freedom grabbing momentum but also something more boring. It filled my mind with potential and perversion as madness closed in to the desolate clocks, which stand in rows; solitary,

silent, in penitence for their awakening. Song in the key
of concrete:

Even if you offered me a ticket to Jesus
Close to the golden dawn
Around dragonfly hills
Above the treasury of the girl
Who dreamt of fairies
Why would life insist on dragging me down?
Don't look so scared
this is just a passing complexion,
One of my bad days.
To achieve imitation of the birds
Why would I like spiralling around and around and
around?
Circling wheel with fuzzy boundaries
A mere spectator circling
Through an ordinary day
Song in the key of concrete
Would you like to watch a film?
Or slip into bed or something?
Or contemplate the silence?
So here's what's happening
I've got to deal with you
Don't care your life away
Finding out why the tangent breaks
If I said what I really thought
would you like to call the cops?
Do you think it's time I stopped?
Why are you running away?
Above the scrapbook of memories
A train of thought-driven purpose
Take a chance by aeroplane
A snapshot in an album
Let gravity seek help
And kiss me
For if the circle breaks

I'll spill the beans
Soft on the inside.

    We want to kill pain with pain- so that suffering is certainly real. The temptation is to blame all those who have built us up and provided the building blocks for confusion leading to classic traits such as Oedipus complex or violence against those trying to help. *For from within, out of the heart of man, come evil thoughts, fornication, theft, murder, adultery, coveting, wickedness, deceit, licentiousness, envy, slander, pride, foolishness. All these evil things come from within, and they defile a man* (Mark 7:20). That you cannot carry fire in your clothes without burning them is perhaps a fleeting example of God trusting us a little too far for we are often without the assent of sin, and so closer to redemption than we think.

If I could dream
Without a single silken petal
Falling on my body
Tempted by a moistless breeze
Impassioned by a soulless tale
I would swallow my pauses
To pass through
Civilization's ladder
Of motley myrrh
Shadow and filigree
Like steam
Beams the dewdrops gently
Seem
As the ventures gather
But a vat of jam
On a bed of green thyme
Indoor fireworks
And fishermen mystically singing
Along the shore
"Relax ye sweet codfishes"

The finer points rather dulcet
Strained from a particular vernacular
The spoken word exhausted-
Where did all the lilies go?
Crispened by the falling light
Dread the night that they may soften
Wank your pollen forth
Infect the highest sect
Wrapped in tightest cellophane
A fly is being formed
Uglier than pillar catapulted mush
Drunker than the sound of karaoke
Still I ponder words once said
To mean some truth
Are but blasphemed pomegranate cries
Uncouth
Stay shy my dear
Bleak never meant to do you any harm
Daybreak my mood rocks back
A single raindrop impact
My might is here
No bars are open
They are all at work
Empty escape
Perhaps I should root myself
Watch my nails erupt
Sway
Dream of killing time
Making love to the sky
Where I belong
As the points blather
But a drug to the manic man
Just passing through
On my way to somewhere more civilized

It is often told that it is the cure which is the
frightening thing and certainly the idea of being
sectioned and living with a bunch of depressives,

queens, manics, suicides, psychotics and the plain evil is not sensible but to be a madman. But when madness is mixed with innocence things get slightly strange. The citadel moves its shadow to the forum of fools, three years unconscious to the wall, spread like a gland in the ether. A moronic laugh ensues, like mortar in the distance, all centred on our provisions. Every opportunity but no potential. Doctors have made the mysterious aspect of madness disappear; where people were once seen to be supernatural it is just another aspect of their illness. Another invented disease. The doctors who hold themselves to be shaman have taken the power. People take advantage of weakness. Has it not been said that you should cling to faith for we must strive manfully; custom is overcome by custom and if thou knows how to let men alone, they will gladly let thee alone to do thine own works.

I will be the patient said the saint in the waiting room. I will be the sugar in the tea. I will be the child in the destiny. I will be the spanner in the works. But I will never tell a confounded stranger anything except my name rank and number. I will be the cross in the tattoo. I will be the taint in the blood for you I will be there for you but- Nothing changes by staying the same- If you can't beat them join them- Don't shit on your own doorstep- Flowers are like faces- Genius is close to idiocy- Cleanliness is next to godliness- What is harping on about wealth without happiness- You cannot carry fire in your clothes without burning them- Why fight a losing battle. What is the point of dissonance?

Psychosis is driven by futility and is a radical expansion of the theme. What is the point of psychosis? It is driven by boredom and is expansion of the mind trying to retrieve control. *Men have called me mad, but the question is not yet settled whether madness is or is not the loftiest intelligence, whether much is glorious, whether all of it is profound, does not spring from disease of thought. Those who dream by day are cognoscente of many things that escape those who dream only at night.* (E. Allen-Poe) The greatest scientists, inventors and artists often followed patterns of strange behaviour. To think up something new you have to be a little touched. Is genius that close to idiocy? Both in the world and asylum the real outlet for psychosis is hysteria but far too often it is by the chemical.

Robotes was a strange fellow, a Greek by birth and such a brain on a man that he was incapable of becoming the pilot he promised as he was always thinking to the point of distraction. He joined squadron 56 in his youth and was the standby pilot to break the sound barrier. As a civilian he studied medicine and became an eminent genetic psychiatrist. He ended up working at Claybury mental asylum after a disgrace involving dehumanizing experiments in genetic cloning which went rather too far. He carried on these experiments on the unfortunate inmates of the asylum. I first met him through my father in 1982. He came round to our house with excited speech and froth on the corners of his mouth such was his excitement at being part of the experiment of Mr Honity to break the time barrier. If this was the psychiatrist what would happen to my father I thought? My father was lately open to conspiracy theories and he obviously had interrogated my dad on this point I thought. However he had more in store for me and after the light of madness had filtered down to me I met him again when I was sectioned in 1991. I remember seeing a social worker that sectioned me on account of my eyes, which were to all evidence depressed. I wasn't depressed I was angry and helpless at being there. Depression is sadness mixed with the despair where things are truly beautiful

Gazing past peaks
I sit I glide
When do you go home?
Unknown
I wander with you along a cold unwelcomed fear
My dear or not
A silent scream rings in my tears
And on and on
Till you I face
Unshared embrace
Defeats the truth
That we once were so bravely fond
Show me where the daffodils grow
Might I ponder spring's sweet glow
Fondling nature's silent woe
Alas this time is done
Lead me to the lily pond
There to speak of heart's beyond
Dare not I stroke my gleaming bond?
For fear of truth unknown
The owl hoots on a mournful blow
That chordless, distorting crow
And mighty sacrifice the show
In memoriam

The nettle ointment stings. Angel'rain hated the sickening reliance on chemicals- "Medication makes a hole in your heart then seals it as a bubble in your blood stream. Fucking nightmare without the acid party. Conifers in a row darting. Angel delights that aren't dissolved. Road close up at 90mph. I am under the car. Face two inches from the floor. All is spinning, spinning, drunk but no drink. "Drink, drink you bitch!" The median triad- it's attacking too fast. No! On the brink. No! Heave. Nothing. Scared! Music-dance-faster. They disallow my imagination. Prescribe mood stabilizer but forget to change the gear to positive. Agitated. Fucked off. Headache. Bastards, the power to play games with brains. Suppress, suppress! All I can write is fucking harmony exercises. I know that harmony will remind me of this place, or rather this place will remind me of harmony. If there were ever a tune to my life, then in its abundance, sleep takes over dreams in the calm of nonchalance. Creature comfort is my wish though I recognise the luxury problems that pass as nightingales sing over the din."

I will own up to hysterical happenings, the laugh left of centre, off the circular, pretty ways beneath death mask in the hallowed ground of graveyards sketched etched pathways of the stealthy vampire of assertions from a congregation of fools in coercion with paranoia that persuade people to take off their hat to entrance with ugliness the panic, the illusion and illumination outside my reality- turn me mad to save me in, forgetful of disparity, hilarity, cruelty and depravity. I hear the nightingale above the din and pay for forgotten sin but I will never tell a confounded stranger anything but my name rank and number. I would believe in ghosts flying, so tough to be away from, above the positivity in crying, among spiralled engrained beauty of fairy beds at sunrise to relax by fireside wooden seats while crowing butterfly-black eyes of deer compete with owls at darkness to peer and peek at teenage glances askance of love in abandonment of cheery hellos and enlightenment of vampire tooth and salty pride of olive skin and yesterdays unknowns. To see a ghost, graded laced chaste reclining in your hair my daring care full of river and sky, hill and high, moonfaced of midnight- that turns me sane to save me in, but I will never tell a confounded stranger anything but my name rank and number.

Do you dare solitude? To try to sea sense you could be lost for years, stuck in a temple close, catch mussels in a net, combine notions like the water stretching sanity to supply duration, like a wave that never returns. Start with imagined antlers of deer as pride. Half hold a temple pastiche to abhor the visibly overwrought and chase the pragmatic soul of the plot, quiet mover persecuted over greensward but you can't thresh the snow like belladonna to the sleeping port.

The smell of guilt
The taste of courage
The heat of the argument
The spark of passion

The fusion of thought
The pain of diversion
The taint of the image
The scar of belief

The trick of time
The death of the lie
The march of the tribute
The ripening of loneliness

Psychosis shatters the mirror on the line of past present and future and I fear I will die by its bright dagger as I entered the corridor of the asylum quite calm and sat down resigned. Resigned that I would be taken to HQ central. Be debriefed and see Robotes. I was quite relieved. I was in a monumentally gothic towered complex of wards and lino lined corridors next to a consulting room and I could hear screams and sighs coming from it. Not great but calm and thoroughly resigned to giving up all the information to the man who had orchestrated the plot. During these hours I was given an EEG, which I assumed, was to take a picture of the brain that had broken the time barrier for experimental data. I sat in the corridor as a stream of his experiments, which I suppose were meant to make me more secure, were paraded in front of me. And I always did like happy endings. A huge girl, obviously a mistake, kept asking me questions about everything and what school I went to and such. She was convinced she knew me, looked totally like a girl I had got off with which turned my best friend against me when I was 16. I later found out she had thyroid trouble but she was then just a fat version of a girl who had turned my best friend against me which Robotes had conducted.

Rolling over in the clover
Over the white cliffs of Dover
The worm alighted upon
 A butterfly I see
The one who sits upon the leaf of the tea
Those resplendent wings as a kite
Bountiful travellers of the air
Whose regalia so bright
A travesty of beauty
I behold from the light grass
And spied a grasshopper
Rubbing his arse
How do I get the wings to stretch?
Upon the winds and fetch
A travesty of beauty
Far from myself this wretch?

This is easy said the grasshopper
Jump into the web
For the spider will encase you and ebb
Your life away to change
And decide as he did lie
Preparations to fly
A travesty of beauty
Cocooned within the spider's eye.
Days went and weeks went by
And the spider attached
Wing of bee and feeler of ant
One day appearing with glee
From silk and web
A butterfly emerged from head to knee

A travesty of beauty
A merge of ant and worm and bee.

Yet to that worm as he lay
Upon the tea leaf so gay
Was his life's reward
A morbid imitation of nature's hoard
A travesty of beauty
Far too far from delight's cord?
A fabrication of the three insects
He was
Neither one nor the others cause
He took on each ones ugly absurdity
He was a meaningless entity
A travesty of beauty
Parody of wanteefly in a word.

      In my naivety I thought he was going to show me all the details of the plan and that I was the missing piece of the mind map, moisture affected, the conclusion to a book flicked over by the greatest minds in history- and written by Mr Honity, but I got what I paid for now whistling past the graveyard. Why does it take the tears of a woman to see how men are? Loneliness is too overwrought and salty pride brings you down to the depths of depression lingering in the circle of solitude. The moon was given to illusion and watching warring smirks selling pain, I latch onto the smitten characters whose faces crack with the frost. I'm too young to die by your dagger bright mirror. Plaster hoisted onto the oracle to catch beauty moving in hotel expression to find style other than this creeping madness. Still introspective time to explore gravity and sublime hysteria. Do I trust myself? Or am I too reliant upon the reflection of others and good times spent in the outside safety of the hospital's grounds.

Long shadows over pastures neat
Bottomless forests deeper sink
Sweet smell of earth
I stroke the sky
With thirsty eyes
That blush with pride for you
Lush grass, lush scene
With sheen complete
Clasped buttercups in fallen heat
Inspired the caterpillar
Who climbing his brief
stops
To bask in your beauty
Living creatures large and small
Bide their moments here
And so refreshed in sense and thought
I can't compare

Anyway I waited all night for him to come out of his room but he never did. Instead more creatures from my life appeared as signs of his genetic bungling until I was given a couple of injections, which I assumed were truth drugs. I took them as stoically as I could and they made me stare for days so much so that I could not speak to a friend who visited and they slowly numbed the psychosis from me until I couldn't see why. Maybe I got it right first time. Anyway I continued to smoke for the next twenty years and it took me half a one to get out of that hole. My uncle could have done it with half a cigarette but I'm afraid to tell you that I meant half a year. Claybury rejects.   Maybe it was filled with the rejects of a mad scientist after all! An angel of the rain approached an inner room and perched herself gently on a plastic chair. There she listened with beated wing:
Consultant: Well, you've made a complete arse of yourself this week you stupid cunt. Get the fuck out of here. You are trying to make a mockery of us all- and at your own expense! Well isn't that considerate of you.

You silly bitch! Ten other highly intelligent superiors snigger. They sit in the ring at which I am present. All look approvingly at the consultant (for their own benefits).

Consultant: So you wanted to die did you or was that diet? (Others snigger, one almost uncontrollably) Here you are bitch, take this knife in front of this audience present and do it- go on do it. Liked being shunted up the cunt did you - liked this life, liked enjoying others, did you? Oh, I'm wasting my breath. In fact I can't believe I even bothered to waste my time on scum like you- get the fuck out of my sight.

Others: Here, here huh huh huh. The consultant seethes and proceeds to carve her like a spit roast.

Consultant: Diet wasn't it? Oh sorry did I get it wrong, ha ha ha ha. Consultant goes to prod her. She grabs the handle of the professional grade carver with serrated edge and does them all in one swipe from left to right (including the occupational therapist which was a pity, she did try, but then she shouldn't have made me sit through a pissing art session, bitch- and the best minimalist cubism I produced- no fucking respect).

Wasted and wounded my fetish was to leave this place as his life gave up the ghost. Ardently I walk the boards brooding for under lanterns skywards maybe a berth for two in Chinatown, a red saffron gown of St George killing the tolerance is like a throat dry from talking, a distraction I would endure to preserve adventure alone. Toughen up and face up to versatility. I was turned around. Loneliness, like wisdom, treads a thousand stars to a ride of grace and leaves no print but is a personal fantasy, which joins the will of Victorian seclusion with the phantasmagoria of madness. Those mortals who are near death now control the raven. Once I had a feeling of psychosis or should I, say he had, me because you can't really control your covenant from this curious whole calling. A kingdom for a voice. Psychosis is to be acted upon. It takes away the responsibility so that you can no longer sin. To each their own is the point reached by loneliness that can propel onwards and upwards but for whose benefit? "Like scum at least you rise to the top" I said to Angel'rain. "They fuck you up to fuck you up" her expression seemed to say. But really to go to the depths of one's soul is to find enlightenment and to believe that voice from above, as the reason why one is alive is to truly give thanks. I remember the words of Joy Division's Atmostphere. Don't walk away in silence.

Chapter 5 Between the Candle and the Flame

It made me feel so confident to be in contact with a secret confidant and decisions could be factored by what he would have done. Given a certain situation there was a certain response that Michael would have given. Like being suddenly animated about something, like a steadfast opinion or calm way of reacting to some given situation, like the space between the candle and the flame. Responsible, reliable, English, reckless, astute, steadfast, traditional these all spring to mind. How would a fighter pilot deal with a situation? Sometimes I would wait for the synchronicity to kick in and be in reality just a drunk. Like an actor it was easier to deal with your weaknesses and it took time to perfect the art of just responding. It wasn't easy to explore his character as the family only talked about him occasionally and it was contended that I should not become like him. I got into motorbikes and planes as a matter of course and I played the part. Eventually it was like an instinct honed to the right decisions when right. It had the meaning that everything was guaranteed and it could lead to good decisions. It made choices simpler in a certain way. It made me mean what I said and speak from a contrite heart. I stared at the candle alight and all these things came to pass. I would have little symbolic successes, which I would call missions, and go to my local pub to have a pint. "One of those roles that get you through" I said to Angel'rain.

I stumbled upon his suitcase memorabilia at my Grandparents house when I was 18. I suddenly realised that he had reacted and responded to intense pressures reliably all his life. Quite a thing to live up to and only 5 years to do it by! Still I had Doris Day, our secret love to rely on. The only thing I had heard of him was when I leant my head out of the car window on a daytrip as a child and my dad said I would end up like my uncle. My mum and grandparents seldom talked about it through their grief at seeing him shuffle the mortal coil back in 1953. His gift was the gift of memory and we have spoken of him with family members since:

Take thou the gift and hold it close and dear;
For gifts that die have living memories--
Voices of unreturning days, that breathe
The spirit of a day that never dies. (Prometheus)

You see it is all part of the way we think. According to what is expected of us, for glory, entertaining people, doing what is right, reacting according to culture, emotional framework, past triggers. In spectral diversity we are allowed to have different perspectives. We all see the colours differently. What might be explained is green to me might not be green to you but is our understanding of that hue. We all share the same cultural and emotional ways but differ in our expression of these perceptions. No two people are the same and this should be respected. Just because you think you are the reincarnation of a fighter pilot and spend your days dressed in military jackets, or are convinced that heaven failed through grief and believe in just getting on with it, it does not make your perspective any less valid than the man who likes birds, football, gambling and fighting down the pub. As long as you are not hurting anyone by your actions then your framework of seeing the world fits into spectral diversity.

The crux of the matter is how does one cope with fear? I generally see it as dealing responsibly with situations, being reliable, having a conditioning by knowing it will be ok, steadfastness and the willingness to experiment with danger. In many ways it is a way of keeping one's nerve in difficult situations that is the lynchpin of anxiety. Hence its relevance to me. For instance faced with verbal threats or deprivation such as mind numbing drugs in hospital. It is amazing the stand you can take when you have the feeling of a military presence in your thoughts. Like your dad says it gives you backbone. Especially with my dad being missing for long periods of my teenage years it gave me a role model. Unfortunately this role model was quite rebellious in his way and stood for tradition but also for a sense of experimentation and recklessness. The really scary emotional parts of life need to be embraced in much the same way as the charge to fight an enemy in flying. It becomes like a honed instinct to survive and prosper and ultimately to care for God, Queen and country. It is the feeling of being brave that eventually filters through one to cause acts of valour in a disappointingly unchallenging world as it is today.

It became an expression of what I thought about the world and how it had changed for the worse in the past 50 years with the onslaught of progress, gender and economic shifts. The meaning of being a man, or English for that matter. Definitely it replaced that in-built path of just reacting by how you were brought up. I often looked at my hands and thought how similar they were to his in the gap between the candle and the flame. This made me feel proud, and if there was a master plan, it was the mystery that I could have been designed specifically for this. I think progress is as much about imagination as actual bravery. *Anything that one man is capable of imagining, other men will be capable of making a reality.* (Jules Verne)

How much is being a mad dog useful in combat? It's better to burn out than to fade away. Obviously controlled madness is useful as fury and tenacity and certainly many fighter pilots may have had the manic energy to sustain them. There nothing quite as convincing as a manic-depressive in full swing. However the RAF deals with madness by encouraging virtue, discipline and responsibility in their pilots. I would not be able to join the RAF for example because of my diagnosis. It is not just a wild sense of adventure and pure talent that makes a skilled pilot. Hence sensitivity is recognized. However it is the catch twenty-two that says you have to be mad to fight in the first place and only if you are not mad are you truly mad.

How much was it a way to stability? The easiest way of explaining it is to look at the simplest form of engineering. When clockwork is in balance everything functions as it should. A little weight here, a minute reorientation, a little oiling there sustains the equilibrium and hence the function of the watch or mind or aircraft. A clockwork system is that which should sense conditions and perform a level of balance that is directly linked to the inputs. The system in an aeroplane is really a set of input/output devices that synthesize modest control requirements. The watch is a spring, which is suitably released by a set of cogs turning a wheel in increments to tell time. Both are in stability and balance. This follows that they should be simple- what is a simpler monitoring system than clockwork? In a watch it provides increments to predict time. In an aircraft the simple clockwork-hydraulic features provide linkage between pilot and control. Care will be taken to create a feedback error loop in the control system to minimize pilot attention so that their only significant workload will be in overspeed conditions through four subsystems- engine control, primary flight controls, secondary flight controls and utilities to provide for the carefree handling during the performance flight envelope. The fuel control unit which is a hydro-clockwork device mounted on the engine measures engine parameters and gives just the pilot the feel of the throttle for optimum efficiency over the wide range of speed, altitude, temperatures and acceleration. Through a closed loop control system elevators, rudders, ailerons and secondary flight controls such as flaps, slats, spoilers and airbrakes can be conventionally arranged with rod and pinion gears which at their simplest are either used or unused. Signals have to be passed as feedback to the control avionics. Avionics have to be designed for all six degrees of freedom and designed for stable, carefree manoeuvre especially for take-off and landing and for hydro-mechanical assistance to have a degree of autostabilisation. The watch keeps balance. The pilot feels the controls and the airplane hence responds. Engineering is a reflection of how our minds work since it is often said that the mind is a tool to create tools to make life easier. How engineering completes the feedback loop, which is essential in making the right decisions, is known as imagination in the mind through the feedback loop of logic. We find the space between illusion and illumination between the candle and the flame.

How much was it a way of forming positivity? I think it was a way of dealing with disappointment. After all we had been flying like angels for two generations so what did it matter if I did not achieve? It let me concentrate on the majestic imagination. Negativity ebbed away through the knowledge that my uncle was part of me. From this perspective I experimented with LSD and had conceptual notions above my station. From teenage years I would try to expand my experience within. Being basically introverted it had appeal to dwell on the mind's wonders at a young age. But my personality is a consequence of many variables. Having been through psychology the strategy is to rid yourself of extreme thoughts and negativity such that you can live the life you have. However what if you could live the life you wanted to live? To provide for positive thinking by use of ego generating memories to enhance your ability to think straight.

When I am anxious and trying to achieve the impossible ego generating memories seem to reverse and cause a confused state where it is vitally important to complete the situation however irrelevant or disjointed they come across. NLP is a process providing a shift from accepting and towards living. Memory selection and imagination are often based on mood. Hence mood is based on imagination and memory selection if this is a perfectly reversible equation (which as thermodynamics theory predicts is often not so simple with the variables involved). Not being afraid to combine our fantasy, manic world, subconscious and conscious brain activity provides positive thinking as described in Jason Peglers book NLP. He talks about how to programme your brain, helps to prove that you can be who you were born to be and to overcome the perceptions of negatives outside yourself. For when I looked in the mirror of a conforming, unconceptualising and materialistic Essex society often I was confused as to whom I was again and perhaps NLP would have helped me with inadequacy and achieve the recognition that characters like Walter Mitty or the rock star in Pink Floyd's the Wall craved. I think actually it is a very common way of spectral diversity to think of flying and all children use it as part of their imaginative growth

Maybe breaking the sound barrier
Sensitive, seldom and sad
Wasn't a Star At All
When rhythmic resonance breaks
The chord of intimacy
The music bears an incantation
From former to now, from land to sea
And fondly the soul we
Always trust in a higher intelligence
Hitler's plan for heaven to extinguish
The darkness of a flare in a light place.
For the spirit is in these chimneyed dreams

Brought into the public domain
That prayer accomplishes
Sees past autumn leaves
Sees past mans achievement
The body waits behind the screen
To where the treetops swing in the breeze
To where the eyes look serene
To where my hopes galore pinnacle and spiral
Wantonly fermenting the brew of my form
Now the ear has frequented
The beautiful new dawn
For I am had by the ribbon on your tongue
Sound's noises rattle and hum
The space between land and sea
And time itself perhaps
A tumultuous coven of equinox
The sonic boom was conceived
Reverently creating the blush of honour
The wave of consuming reason
Milk of human kindness
In the clarity of the plan
To win back the valour of heaven
The sound barrier is achieved
Wishes regalia,
Dripping Icarus off snow-laden arms
Able to answer a moments twain
My uncle's slender form
Wished a breath for her flaming gaze
And flew too close to the sun
With beingness of wax and feathers
Appealing to God's nature
A star Child
But from the hand that rocks the cradle
Eternal hope springs
That lushly his breath shelters
Maybe breaking the sound barrier
Sensitive, seldom and sad
Wasn't a Star At All.

Matthew & Lorraine Woods

Chapter 6 True Truant of Memory

Fantasy is a part of imagination. Imagination is always encouraged. Fantasy is made up of perspective and is in turn made up of memory context. Fantasy is a shell tossed in the sea of imagination without the grounding of reality:

A handful of shells
Took fright to the sea
They tossed, they turned
They betwixt, they betweened
Then a huge wave burst
Upon their beings
So high they were caste
Soon landing on deck
In a flurry, they rested
The vessel at anchor

Fantasy overrules reality when brought into play to control anxiety. It takes control when there is a fear of losing what you are or what makes up your world generated by the past existing within the present. Normally the process of memory generation is selective: the ego managing what is selected to introduce well-being into each given scenario, giving a reliable sense of oneself. However bad memories and imagination, remaining in the subconscious, stimulated by anxiety often leads to misinterpretation of perspective. The devil written backwards – lived. Someone who did live but does not anymore. That was how life had become, where layer upon layer of negativity spewed to reveal the side of life that was not what people wanted to hear on a Sunday afternoon. But of value? Yes, I suppose. For those desperate to relate their own anguish in some way is useful for others at a similar point and for those who desired the study of thought. It comes back to conformity. Some may say what is uncomfortable.

Some may wear Goth cloth; others abuse alcohol in a trendy bar in the city. We observed and did pretty much all we could to join the interceders. Until one day, anti success. A few too many pills and I met him on a hospital bed in A and E. Choking on Charcoal preparation and not quite able to get perspective on the room I was in, a man wheeling a hospital trolley wearing an overall came up to me. He offered me a cup of tea and looked kindly. What are you doing here? He continued to tell ways that I would be more successful in doing what I had wanted to do. He continued on his way. Psychosis is a negative term. Medics are only caused to use such a term in negative circumstance. Medic's only deal with ill health, an intrigue of negative webbing of assumption when out of control may trip into the bizarre. Fear sets in when control is lost. I was psychotic about a cat owner once and the next day, I found a mask of a cat next to my outside bin. The unexplainable causes us to panic. The unexplainable running away with itself may be an example of the devil in his best party dress.

The World is psychosis
Bending in the wind
Among smiling faces
The silver snake erupts
A current balmy striking out
Zoom! The jollity is announced
Hissing and rising then falling
Protecting precious hands
Wots a pleasure treasure trove
Among heaven's calling
Pummel and bounce in the light of the sun
To see the life called summer
Fooling tangible atlas catch
And snatch your life is weathered here
First one then another
Hand reaches out

Ting, touch, tinging much of a
Muchy much called muchness
More fun, more fun
Whoosh, twist and spin
Shallow shells and bells and
Rabbits' ears and donkeys' tails
Never to fall to the ground
Never to let hysteria take over
Pressure and shockwaves are overcome
Our world it slithers round and round
And up and down against the wind
So that the sound barrier is broken.

Bad thoughts arising during anxiety reach into your feelings. This is the elation of psychosis. It frees you from anxiety in a perverse way and here lies its appeal. Angel'rain recounted her journeys in the sullen streets. I reluctantly walked to the station. It was freezing and I tripped, bouncing onto a blanket of congealed ears, as I fell, my ears fell too. I could not get up from the slippery scene. A dwarf man casually whistled onto the scene with a wooden box marked 24 and some surgical spirit and as he picked the earrings from the random ears, he looked in my direction and laughed. 'Only nine carat, only use nine carats'. His face was worn with kindness and he looked in my eyes with intense simplicity. The bus was laden with trays of all kinds containing watches, rings, broaches and gems of all sorts. Quite stunning a find this void bus was and I prepared myself for another journey. Yes, it was true; again I was journeying to Hainault but to go another way this time. And where I got on, nobody else dared follow. The engine was off, the smell of musty aftershave wafted through as he approached me, he had undone his door and come to talk to his only customer and then I noticed why - My black gloves had given him license to sell. He introduced me to his wares. 'A fine collection I have here!' He went on to explain... 'When my business went bust I decided to join London Transport, and what could be better than this, setting up my own place here, I only house the finest gold'

.

I couldn't help but find him funny, as usual, my spirits were not high and I found him harmless enough so I decided to play on. My move, and where could I take it now - There was no need, I just let him ramble on and he gradually unfolded himself... 'Now you see, If I had frozen them for you there would have been no pain, I don't like guns they make a funny clinking noise as you use them'. I explained that mine were of the finest 24-carat and gunned at the most reputable jewellers in London. Then he advanced towards me to inspect the damage. His fingers touched my lobes and then a sharp twist was all it needed. He leaned towards me closer, closer and then his buzzer went. 'Well, it was time we were on our way' and he mounted his chair, smoothed his big wheel and the void bus rambled out of Chigwell Row. 'They really suit you, you know, I mean I couldn't imagine you without them now, It's amazing how much they improve an appearance, in fact I could even offer to do you a second pair and then you would look doubly suitable - and I wouldn't hurt you, I can guarantee it' I was bored with this talk now, he was non-character material and not only that I could only hear parts of his speech due to the noisy engine. I decided to agree and disagree at what I considered to be appropriate intervals and also give the occasional smile and nod, he wouldn't be aware and probably was too thick to realize that I didn't want to be bothered with him any longer. I began to sink into my own thoughts, staring at the gold and admiring the amethysts. The vibrations of the bus calmed me, they always do but this time it was different, they were more intense, and as I looked toward tray no 36, the jewels took the form of objects de sex. I liked it and so did he. I saw him laughing, his head wrenched back, he no longer cared for the road, and when he turned I beheld the most enormous jewel I had ever seen, this was his pride and joy, it glinted in the light and he stroked it back and forth, this had been on tray 61, and I had read next to it at the time that it was to be set in the finest gold to become the most incredible specimen on offer. I half wished to see it completed but knew that I would probably not revisit this chapter. The void bus stopped, the doors opened and I walked uncomfortably to Hainault station. I looked at the bus as it shunted past, he hooted and was gone.

Often we behave in society according to our super-ego. The part of you which tells you what you should do. The voices of family, authority or morals. In the 19th century the Salvation Army fought a campaign against prostitution. Whatever its moral implications they saw it as an evil which needed redemption for the victims- often young girls lured to London by promises of work. A great, great grandmother of mine, Elizabeth Cottrill used to take in prostitutes to her home in Whitechapel during the jack-the-ripper era, to save them from their plight and eventually secured the first hostel of the Salvation Army. In her own words 'At the penitent form I took the feather out of my hat and came home like a drowned rat, crying and weeping for joy, and from that day I went forward, not to sing "Rescue the Perishing", but to do it ! For 'I said, "Lord, I'll do whatever you want." One snowy February night a girl penitent asked, "How can I be Christian – the life I'm living?" I said, "You must give up that life." I lived at No. 102 Christian Street, Commercial Road, next door to a pawnbroker's. It was nearly 12, and my husband and six children were asleep. I gave her some supper – coffee and a little bit of cold meat, and bread and butter. I didn't want any myself. I wanted to get to bed. I was full of prayer and thankfulness, thinking about her broken-hearted mother and how glad she'd be. I made her up a bed in the kitchen on some chairs with old coats and dresses – the best I could get without waking the others. I couldn't undress her. She was a clean girl. She had run away from her home near Brighton with another girl, expecting to find London streets paved with gold. They went to the Tower Hill to see the soldiers, imagining they'd find a husband straight away, but only got into trouble. I took her home the next day. I said, "You must ask your mother's forgiveness, and if she won't take you in I'll bring you back." Of course, her mother did take her in, only too thankful to see her safe. After this, the soul-saving work amongst these girls went on, and I would get four and even eight in my little place. So I began to pray for a bigger house.'

This is where the voice from God can do great good but often the super-ego is not so clear and can be a form of well meaning pie in the sky, so that moral indignation can come out during flights from reality and become ineffectual. Some would say that this fervour should be channelled. Activities such as NLP, Christianity or Islam can do this. But what if psychosis in itself can be harnessed? What if these things were really happening? Does psychosis make us act in the nick of time? Outside the yellow streets were busy, my eyes were sore and tired, I wasn't used to being up in the morning after working all night, I preferred to sleep. Today was different, the air smelled particularly full of spring and legs moved easily. I watched and caught the smell of food on the wind. There were many pubs here and it was near to lunch time and this smell was mouth watering, I was hungry and walked almost possessed along the street to buy some chips. I thought that the story of Jesus was being staged in these dingy, crowded streets. A young child and mother were being harassed by a boyfriend and my thoughts turned to them being holy and the man being evil. I confronted the man with argument and as for the scenario just being an argument I turned it as good versus evil. I threw my chips at the man whose countenance was pure anger and walked off singing Nirvana. I have thought of vans as parked to abduct people and convinced a whole shop that this was happening or thoughts that kids were playing football with heads leading to severe dread, an embarrassing event where I stopped a football match because of this psychotic thought. Situations based on anxiety lead one to misinterpret what is happening; to feel like a scarecrow in society' midst. But my relative believed that one person can make all the difference to those around them. When is it the time to act? William Booth acted in a time when his ideas were seen as mad.

The madman believes in
The impossible fire
The military many
The friends he knew
Flowing forever
In the corn fields
Old sensations rushing in
Erecting form from
Delicate regions of the soul
Glass cages of the psyche
And fire rushes in
Two spectres like lamps quivering
Living earth spinning a tapestry of light
Where life seems a laugh
And love is telling him to stay
Portraying the elegant rapture
Kindled in his heart
And he starts to burn
Left him bleating here
Everybody burns
Above his head

Society just keeps up appearances where people are content in a shallow way without self-doubt. All good as far as it goes. According to William Booth:

There is a pattern. And there is a pattern in catching and throwing, too. You have to follow the right pattern. Often this is in the form of an evangelical life where you listen to the voice of God. Sometimes it can be the positivity released during NLP. The tap of imagination is heightened by hyper-awareness during the flight or fight experience of anxiety and to block off the thoughts associated with it is pointless.

'Do I plan to de-value the devil?' spake the vole to the hare. 'Well a fine idea I would say. Upon which basis would you conclude? Upon the basis of ever-growing awareness and everlasting faith in God my dear friend. 'Why ever do you care to share your thoughts with a hare? Replied hare. 'A hare is quick to act, quick to the game, quick in mastery, quick in tongue, quick to motion in a motionless void', 'I see' said hare as he spun himself a pirouette 4, 5 times anticlockwise and landed on the sawdust floor in a rather ungainly state. Then he twitched his nose and scratched the behind of his ears whilst scratching his bottom. 'OK vole, you have me intrigued' he added in a peppery manner. 'Should I take minutes on the matter in hand or do we plan for the trees to bear witness?'

'To intimate antiquity would be a vole's consideration, such is a voice to sound my fears dear hare. Close we are to the truth though I fear the closer we strive to be, the farther we are from it. It would have been so much simpler to utter two words 'I believe' at the beginning of time. Proof, proof, proof, evidence, evidence, evidence. Enquiry, debate, showdown, mood-matrix, crunch and disperse. For what? I needed proof of God's existence again and again. Did I enjoy the process? Yes, but sometimes there were huge leaps of understanding undertaken that caused me much pain in order to shed light on the meaning of life.

'I'm sorry my dear fellow, I don't really follow your train of thought!' Hare glanced at a picture of a deformed Mona Lisa mid cubist gaze, hanging from Vole's porch door. 'Your gaze or her state hare, I ask you?' vole went on 'Do I see what you see? Does God see your distortion? Does awareness lead me to absolution?'

Vole came closer to Hare and held his hand shakily, 'Last night hare, I was raped by the devil. I was forced against the wall and held down. I could not move my arms. They were pinned to the bed and I choked as breath was forced out of me. I saw no one.... it happened the month before, and the month before that.

The fear of the nightmare lived as a conscious exploration of my mental overload. The truth played out. You see hare; I have watched those movie chillers. I vaguely recollect the exorcist hype. Such warped creators, how could they imagine such obscenity? But you see the imagination is not so imaginative after all. Within the realms of imagination is mere tragedy or jollity transpiring. Feigned stories of the bat drenched night, a vampire's bite, a cat's slow wagging tail.... I prayed, before the event, during, and after the event and those prayers confirmed God's presence. I didn't feel that I could approach anyone on the subject of these strange battles apart from the badger who lived near the sycamore tree. I knew he would not judge me or consider me bad company to keep or even be just scared of me. Contemporary therapy stated that prayer might keep the idea alive. I understood the principle but was not prepared to compromise. How could I settle the debate in my mind? How could cognitive behavioural therapy work side by side with God? They were all I had! And so desperately alone for fear of losing the world mid attack, I thought I was about to lose God too. But hare, you see, perhaps God wanted me to quieten while he faced this business directly for me. The very next time this nightmare scene repeated, I approached it differently - with calm confidence in the Lord, and I allowed God to take over. I knew the foundation of Christianity was there and my belief was strong after confirmation in the kitchen that night months before. I bore these moments with God and each time they replayed, eventually the fear diminished and the devil left my soul. God was victorious. I saw it through as a cat in a vat of boiling water, - and then I returned to his feet. He did not abandon me, I did not abandon him, and I still have not left him.

But of course hare, nice people ought not to mention such things, oh no, they wouldn't dare. Their reputation, their pride, their privacy. Why would I want to be reminded of desperation on a daily basis? 'Look' the forest folk would say 'there goes the violated vole'. But no hare, why do I care to tell you of my dealings with the devil? Hare looked plaintively through vole with wonder. 'It's ok hare, that's why I tell you. It is real, it's ok, it's an episode of brain spill, of shrapnel unleashed. Possession by the devil is perhaps a metaphor for this confused, highly stimulating, frightening adventure of the mind which in my case was a passage of time past that youth could not convert but just held in a pocket waiting to be freed by God who was waiting 'til the time was right. And yet who would dare to add these happenings to a human's condition in the realms of spirituality? Perhaps not just metaphorical notion after all? And now I am here, I can walk, I can talk, I can eat, I can sleep, I can laugh, I can play, I can thank God for his love for me every day. Let it be known hare, nothing is beyond the realm of possibility in God's eyes.

Vole finally sat down in his cosy armchair and rested his eyes for enough time to remember what he was going to have for supper. He cleaned his whiskers and prepared himself to experience the mirrorscape again during the night to come. He was aware that after bringing the subject to their attention, the events might want to replay. 'Let it go' he uttered under his breath. '.... To God' continued hare.

The two held each other's backs in a loving yet semi medical chum hug. The trees grew dim and the two prepared a fire. The fireflies darted and the dragonflies drew speed as the dampening air saw a chill in their cold noses. Vole gathered the vegetables that hare had kindly brought that afternoon to make a stew and the subject gently turned towards things that reminded them of other things. Vole asked hare if he had seen the tree next to the pond that had reminded him of an elephant's foot and Hare chuckled about the sea of autumn leaves that reminded him of a bowl of muesli.

'How beautiful the forest is' said hare. 'Yes, it is', said vole 'We shall live here for our evers'.

The filters of reality are reactions that take thoughts and turn them into a vast wood of emblems of past hurts. Traumas become like edifices of our past reminding us that we have been there before. We wander through the woods sharing our secrets and neuroses. It is important to have perspective on your past but during anxiety these bonds become weakened and hence even when there is no threat; these statue trees play on our mind and become real. Fears raise themselves and we mistrust our environment turning it into a zombie landscape of trees come alive. It is like your memory plays truant during anxiety and you have the overwhelming feeling of confusion- statues of bad memories arise so that your rationale, mood and emotional outlook all become magnified to a point of real threat.

When vole woke that morning, he thanked God that the cycle of trauma had not repeated during the night. As he emerged out of the woods progression was evident. Jesus was evident.

Chapter 7 Enjoy Your Time In Passion's Eye

Time has chosen us to go on and bear fruit, fruit that shall last in our everyday lives, in the things we do, to bear witness to God as we go around living our lives by the example we show to others enough to be returned. To give love and to have it returned is the most important opportunity in life. To use other people as mirrors. For to jump through the portal from the rusting pod waiting room, the zenith of engineering achievement, is to fall in love. To follow a woman down it takes the tolerance of a relationship to realise important pearls of wisdom and intent that we call passion. But the relationship with sound barrier had the spirit's gentler equation imploring one to inspire and regulate time so far. Passion also pushes you further. There are certain people you choose to share your feelings, your life. To share the softness inside. Yesterday's purpose is like a map. Ultimately you share your spectral diversity to form indelible bonds.

I first jumped through the portal in the realms of summer holidays. My first sexual experience was there on echo beach. The grass stains. The fumbling. The ecstatic but scary touches, of the wetness and smells. Tracie was my first joining of souls and perhaps led to this whole journey. For maybe she was the woman in white. The sense of bliss coupled with the sense of betrayal and sadness that my best friend's jealousy and love for her was to upset the gladness that we reached. She was stunning and I never chose blondes again. Such were the scars of my rival and best friend turning on me. She gave me a cross earring and this started the seeds of my faith.

There was a friendship
A companion
To reach the beaches

To reach innocence
Accidentally on purpose
There was the girl
Of blonde and lime green
O, the misfortune
Of a virgin breeze
Too pure to shock a starling's flight
Too light to shudder wisdom's gaze
You wisp through
Beauty unparalleled
Of lips of goldust, innocence
Accidentally on purpose

Then there was the friendship
The freedom of cognition
To climb the glint of cliffs
To listen to music on the beach
And compare dreams
But accidents will happen

So there was the girl
Accidently on purpose seduced
And play your path unseen
You dance through youthful locks aglow
In cities face and fields of green
Hail sweet moment,
Enjoy your time
In passion's eye
The vagaries of youth
It made another reduced, to anger
Accidently on purpose
To violence, the throwing of bricks and mortar
To sulken silences and seething
To wreck a friendship past
Accidently on purpose

My first love was a girl of intense caresses and
distance, secrets and openness, words and dreams.

She remains a sturdy and responsible influence in which our imaginations shared; brief three day rendezvous and yearly correspondence. Obsession, yes, but through her immaculate sense of balance and realness in an increasingly unreal world she made my fears seem ordinary. Time well spent in the greenbelt. Growing up having someone to love strangely made decisions easier to control. Distance does make the heart fonder as closeness exists in separation where desire intensifies the character of love.

There are cobwebs over the Albert Bridge
Time zones of creation
And I am reminded
The theme was sometimes tender
Still there and spruce
Path through which we finger
A sense to hysteric cobwebs
That were born to be together
And raised our eyebrows
Mingling with circumstance
That perhaps we were part of the masters' plan

Her minuet breath to shiver the core
In conversation at Castle Ashby
From the eve of prouder caverns
On the open beachfront of afternoon
Half there and deciding to manifest
As frequent as people walking down our way
Yet we are adolescent in equinox
For we pay to stir your chandelling hand
But not to close over your palm
The natural charm she seeded in soar
Broken web to strike the sky with an acorn

Her beauty was familiar
Like the pole of a star flag placed in her hand
Like the French revolution was not ours

Nor mine for believing in you
Nat-West Midland by torchlight
The world sees her in their frontage
As light imitation of another season
To end the sweep of Oarystes pride
As if we were counting success over separation
Held in our swanlike hands
But love is strange
When I beat upon it now at twenty
We looked at the webcore in exile
By torchlight it appears
The miliscention of your mother's wisdom
On enthusiasm, confidence and compromise
Because if a boar could fly
It'd be caught in the web
As romantic as discerned
Like a miracle at Lords
Because if I remember
You did not like cricket or Yamamoto
Or adverbs as an article
So when we have ground beauty to dust
Remaining by your words
Why wish for the moon
When we have the stars.

Then the schooltime romance. Vast summers that never ended. It is strange to think that the vagaries of youth could be so tied up with the summer sun. But they always ended with the onset of winter, like the blooms of summer or bloomers in a spin cycle. We met at sunrise in passion spent at Glastonbury. We shared our fears with a pact not to share neurosis with anyone else. To be lost halfway up a tree uplifted by heady days of wonders untold, moonstruck gravity, St George and the roses.

Thou art the fountain of art
Freely let me take of thee

If you've sucked in your words already
I've saved mine too
I'm still a lot like the past
Stuck in glass cages
Heaven only strikes twice you know

Chose to feel as a small boy
Lining his ideas with pearls
Furled in harlequin blue
Commemorating dreams of sharp whims
A butterfly in being
Padded coal seams
When you've pinned but not out murmured
The only way is up and out.

Prejudice when people affect credibility
And the prickly prejudice, a nightly rose
Will feel your love for the inside
But innocence in her charitable belief
Gets there first
Fear over time relatively
Like a deer the quickest flew
What if heaven should fail?
Springs disclose in my heart
Rise to all eternity.

The real thing is love but heard above the din in an asylum it takes on the form of escape and mixed with catholic certainty and guilt during days of cooperation and indifference it gradually bore the mark of tainted love. Promises of tempestuous love can never last through such painful experiences.

Champagne booms another June
The chameleon's colours rippling beneath
The transparent turquoise sea
Dustless as the virtue which changes thee
So that all that remains of our summer skin

Is shimmering as heat from the sun.
There are echoes of salvation
In the expensive days
In natural ways
To peel the glad tidings out
Of which are taken in haste
Butterfields and strawberry sunsets
Green glades lead to Benfleet cries
Illuminating moondances to swell the skies
And I am me-
Where will you be?
None to hold me
Make undone what has been made
Shake up love
To the big shaken fade
Fill up with gladness
Hope it won't seep away
Bottle it up! Shake it up!
Champagne booms another June.

After the passions are aroused and numbed by
one-night stands, married trysts and trysts with the
indifference, the return to the gothic northern girls of
youth- shapely legs, dancing, dreams and depression.
Loneliness and problems making the life less ordinary.
We were really just making the most of our desperate
theatrics- like a drawn out ballet.

While Cinderella mends her dancing dream
I wake up with pride not braveness
Can the truth be told by an equation?
You said you prefer films to persuasion
Billy Munster watches Betty Blue
As you recall when Harry met Sally
I've been waiting here years but I haven't met her yet
The rabbit I've known as Flibbertigibbet
Is overcome by the darkening net

While Cinderella mends her dancing dream
They've pulled down the cafe where we used to meet
The bombed out buildings are my feelings of rejection
Firmly compounded by loyalty in perfection
For yet another apocalyptic air display
Elequise lightening does aerobatics
And you insist upon standing up with your Rubicon
Lost in remembrance of you bare
All occurring at the same time somewhere
Is overcome by the darkening air

While Cinderella mends her dancing dream
You ask if your crutch is like Egypt
For when you leave like that
It's quite timeless
Like fragments of a rollercoaster
Seamless
Your kisses mock your friends
Endearing, concise and gullible
The man who was paint on the ceiling
Talked of leaving but stayed,
I talked of staying but left
Are their nipples not their brains?
I can't answer your tragical questions
Through the mists and visions of time
But I keep a secret regard
That our ivory tower
Was my secret love for you?

So it was that the dawning and realisation of love flowed between us as we walked along echo beach. Reality is made in love and it is often referred to as having a guardian angel for it affects softness on the inside, which suits closer bonds and invariably creates new life, our daughter Elehail. Was Michael our guardian angel? In him passion abounded. Could it be that God's promise was lived out to wonders everlasting?

Through apportioned light
The angel's flight
Thrown emotion,
Crumpled to kinship breaks
On thoughts of intimacy
The mind finds as imagination
True feelings of closeness
Antiphony of splendour
Carved riches beauty
By an angel's wing
You are thinking
From the hideaway
Of a secret garden.
Then when soft tulips
Open to the virus breaks
Hark a patter of daffodils
Within steady grasp
The heir of intimacy
The body sees as imitation
True art of closeness
By an angel's wing
You are guided
Ever to flow
Through the truth of humankind.
Then when the gleaming sparkle breaks
The beauty of intimacy
The eyes see as a realisation
True vision of closeness
By an angel's wing
You are precious
And to all evidence and investigation
An angel.
Then when valentine yonder breaks
The communication of intimacy
The soul alights as revelation
True grace of closeness
By an angel's wing

You are shielded
From the rain
By my love.

Trust is the key to an extraordinary existence; the grounding, which keeps you happy, and so maybe we should trust in God and know that love is guided by angels. It is certainly a miraculous thing that is not entirely explicable. One cannot truly fall in love through madness. For love is not madness. No *it is sublime sanity through another person's eyes for when we have found our partner, we are not only linking our lives to another individual, we are also entering a myth that reaches far into the most meaning-giving areas of the heart. The happiness we hope for in marriage is a catchall word that embraces many spoken and unspoken wishes for fulfilment. In a sense, the person we marry offers us an opportunity to enter, explore, and fulfil essential notions of who we are and who we can be.* (Thomas Moore)

Spirit's wonders everlasting
Bright and twinkling to Jesus
But the journey of our souls
For our love is like moonglow
Companions for one another
Shall become one flesh
Like a splendid family tree
Its fronds beseech a happy home beneath
A marriage so full
Of joy that angels do fly
Potential made in the hearts of two people
The enjoyment of sense and reason
Full of consistency and trust
Be happy and glad as we approach
The most natural state
Union of two hearts
The weaving together of strands

By angels wing
Upon a windswept apogee
Of earths great livery
And spread our meteor plumes
Rising by God's secret sap
A gentler constancy implores us
To inspire and regulate time so far
To look together for the whole love enchanting
Shared for all eternity
Spirit's wonders everlasting.

Reality is made in heaven. Or so we are led to believe. Whenever we are losing our way then we have to return to its path. If we fall into the arms of another then we make reality from the space between a man and a woman, which stops off from time to time. Since trying to live an isolated existence I have been governed by the space in relationships. Who's to say what a relationship governs? It is often when we lose it that we realise what we've got. It is the space between the candle and the flame. In a previous book I explained it as the chrysalis time. A time lapse between the candle and the flame was a place for words and experiences of the triumphs of love and ages, and inside the renewal of compassion and outside the depiction of stasis wrapped in ages present. Inner ways and outer horizons in the wrap of a heartbeat.

I sip my tea and forget to breathe
I pillage my rest
Cupid's lost bow
Has pierced my heart
I hear the tick
And betray the tock
For delight is had
Living for future memories

The blazing sun many moons on reminds me of how I burnt from inside out once. What's it called again? Spontaneous combustion? A mix of too much medication and high anxiety caused me to seriously overheat to the point that it felt hotter than 40 degrees. I was sweating continuously and straining for breath. My eyes bulged like a rat being squeezed until it spilled the truth. Your friend or your neighbour cannot take inner torture away. They sit by and spend a while not quite understanding what it must be like in there. Nobody wants to witness a life that is too much for the senses to sustain. The pain, the blistering heat, of a tortured soul only to be soothed by a calamine God.

I walked back from taking my daughter to school in the same heat today. There was peace. The traffic roared as usual. Smiles were kind and although their journeys were their own there was a glance of understanding from shared experience of some sort. As I walked, a five pence piece glinted at me and for the first time, I walked by without stooping to pick it up. As I did, a little voice said 'see a penny pick it up, all day long you'll have good luck, see a penny leave it be, all day long you're full of glee'. So whose voice was this? I continued my enquiry... God does not do luck and God certainly knows that money is not the answer to a meaningful life. I continued on my way in the affluent area I live with a smile for those who needed it. Many youthly souls in search of new ideas sacrifice their own sanity to do so whilst leading a cranky half-life. (Better a musician than to sit on a refuse tip). Yet by living the ordinary life, a life designed, tried and tested, tweaked and reported as it was written in the Bible for instance finally allows enough freedom for absurd, highly imaginative and spectacular adventures to be revealed to us in a healthy way.

The chrysalis has encompassed us. My hands are firmly on your chest and we breathe as one for fear of tearing the delicate web. A tear rolls down your cheek and I can tell it has multiple meaning (I won't question you now). You sleep and I sing you a lullaby...

So rest now a-while
My valiant knight
For peace is a gift
We never should fight
Slowly one kiss tends to
Blossom and bud
Sleep now so silently
My tender love
The song attracted the sparrows and finches that settled on the tops of the hedges. They decided to join in with their own dawn chorus as each grain of sand falls through the hourglass of hope.

As we looked at the candle the impression was that we were engulfed in a dream and the world was comfort. Yet inside there were flights of fancy, sensations of care and joy and reality in the transference of feeling. Regret was replaced with integrity, awkwardness with composure, and innocence with desire. Development of realisation was the impetus coursing through our veins to delve into different journeys to find the truth like a stay jewel fruiting along the dairy path, chasing the meteor's bloom until the coppiced lagoon, red setted with explosives let our caged hearts linger on behind glass. The starry heart of pearl thrown and crumpled to kinship was the pod of eternity and we would wait awhile together, first and last and always.

And time stood still
My breath frozen
As I try to blow

The dandelion from its puff

The wind beat me
Fragments of seed
Dispersed then flew
To a better year

Too tired to dream
The clouds tell us something
But we're too confused
We can't read their message

We must keep trying
We must stay strong
Calmness breeds eloquence
In a field full of longing

Only by sharing experience are we set free. The actuality of raising a child together could be beautiful. Cherished destiny led as wonderfully feathered to inspirations happenings of sweet beauty that atoned stranger than talent, fascinated devotion and soothed closer than compassion where serious desire wantonly reigns in fulfilment like a rider upon a ground of ability to transpose form and dynamics from instinctive reality to parallel your soul's vantage. If a tree falls in a forest and you are the only one to hear it then reality is not assured. The tenderness I have viewed through the viewfinder of relationships and stood firm against the struggle we have been through was often, in the mission for social inclusion, the only true bond. With the speed of sound it ushers into a relationship, meaning and fulfilment. Reality is the place between a man and a woman where trust replaces love and love like a pearl brings contentment and makes the ordinary extraordinary:

The ordinary
Enduring in our stead
Our cherished destiny
Gathered on a bed of cotton
Heather your veil
Water flows underneath
Flowers tenfold on hills of old
The swans rose above
Countryside flowers beckon
Murmur what is said
From a heartbeat
A transparent bloodred thread
Dark innocence envelops
Sublime scarlet secrets spent
Gathered from the seabed
In linen,
The extraordinary pearl.

We venture into the valley of mist. I see the particle mist in every dawn, a rising splendour. Green earth I tread where those have died. We touch the bright coloured lights that adorn us with a gentle passion. Yet alive, ghosting the cool air. I fill your eyes with hope that I can only smile upon. The moon was sad that night; a sullen glow fell heavily upon our hearts. But we saw nothing but true happiness in his telling soul. A cockerel cries his plenty and a field is torn by his wish, my dreams fall to heaven and yours rise in reverence to that lowly place for what is higher than this time. For I, the jaunty stag wisening, strutting careful foot forward, is painless and free for I fly like the wind. Forever we will climb together through sun, moon, noon- where seldom a creature has altered, pallor of knowing, pallor of peace overruling. Soft ears, so soft to touch, listen to silent vows, and pray upon each secret shared. They hear my soul, my wrongs, and my rights. Red lips speak in truths that separate the stars and moons and kisses emanate in trust, they burst with vigour, burst with lust. Blue eyes look beyond. They see each smile; they feed each gaze, through a haze of lasting love out of the youthly wild and into the wise woods. We will succeed until the very end when our hearts are tired of this life. In a bluebell wood we will dance as three before time is done. Stars will shine for us then and mine will shoot, always to be in your light. Eve was supposed to be fecund and it is a truism that heaven creates the love of a good woman. You only have to love one woman for one day to be sure of that.

Matthew & Lorraine Woods

Chapter 8 Seeing the Wood for the Trees

Society's answer to mental health, other than vague gestures towards community has never been clear. It lies with empowerment of users and those who have wisdom to deliver souls from a society that sees mental health as dangerous and materialism as self worth. It is not to be insane to feel the spirit moving inside us and most issues are felt by all. Perhaps it is our twisted answer to utopia, which is to blame within our hectic capitalism, which makes vulnerable those whose insight through extended sensitivity is seen as worthless throughout a spiritual journey. In other cultures those with visions are seen as shaman, those with insight eccentric. Perhaps it is the reaction of those around you rather than actual madness that prevails. Those who feel the weight of life could have a voice in society so that we should satisfy our duty to see the suffering in the less protected; the idea of seeing the suffering of Christ indicated in the heightened awareness of mental health. The treatment for a mentally ill patient should be a treatment of loving care, tenderness and kindness, in order to help us cope with our imaginary world, perceived as an enemy, a world in which we often drown. We need help through the woods of insanity

Society should establish, in the education systems, solid emotional foundations that help to work out clear and stable horizons, to be followed for a lifetime. It should be aware of the system of values underpinning the whole human life and make reference to it, especially to avoid that mental illness is lived with anxiety, sadness and desperation. It could fight against relativism, consumerism, pseudo-culture of instinctive desires and pansexualism. It could promote the dignity of mentally ill patients. Society provides stability and confidence. The more you succeed, the more you are bolstered up and the more people believe in you, the safer you feel. Alternatively if you are forever told you have something wrong with you the downward spiral of confidence prevails. Together with being in a poor area and amongst people with low self esteem so the cycle continues. Low self worth is a symptom and cause of mental distress and is self-depreciative. Confidence and high self worth is an alleviation of mental distress and self-appreciation. Community should foster a healthy development of the child, including his brain functions. It should make awareness programs on mental illnesses for the society so that people may know about them and prevent them. Groups whose charisma it is to take care of these patients should not to waver in their commitment and to dedicate particular care to them, given the particular emergency that this illness presents. Be aware of the fact that the rehabilitation of a mentally ill patient is a duty of the whole community together, within the context of solidarity that shows preference for those who are most in need (notes taken from a sermon by Catholic bishop).

Do not be afraid of changing the viewpoint from commonly held panaceas. One learns to prove oneself through personal success and not the way society perceives it. Between those who conform and those who rebel, is the need for integration with society. Everything has its price after all. The most expensive thing society has is the golden bin lid. I was a clear thinker. I schemed of what society's conscience could take to the maker. The golden dustbin lid diatribe above my bed was a circle, condensed in a wheel in a sphere, in a globe within a spiral- it was society's muse. It was the oldest thing I had ever seen. It was the newest thing I had ever touched. It was society's mantle. It stood for the relationships between people, the fragility of consumerism- that some people get left on the garbage heap whilst others rise to the top like scum. Everything would one day cease to exist. Everything had its price.

To boost my confidence I get in touch with psychosis and the ego finds a place in fantasy if not reality. This just polarizes society further when people do not relate with you. Anyone can have mental health issues so importantly why do people see themselves as strange? People are so often seen as judgmental by mental health users whereas mostly it is just people trying to cope with the same problems and pressures you are having. I mean it is not the man dressed in the long trenchcoat looking slightly depressed or the man who chooses to dance through a pub in a green tutu that you have to worry about but the person who appears so normal but is really just riding roughshod over people in their search for more at any cost. Why should we smother aspects of mental health just to fit in, which give such wonder to the inner self and yet reward perversion of the truth through materialism's luxury? Society has many hidden agendas. It is the way we treat society that determines our perspective on mental health and the way society treats us that provides our outlook. Do not become lost in the woods.

Our perceptions of society are all important to combat the causes of anxiety, depression or psychosis for don't blink because access to illness is not exclusive nor the solutions extensive. There are coping strategies that do not mean simple avoidance. One can shut down our awareness as a short-term option. One can provide for shortcomings and identify the creation processes involved to compartmentalise or simplify them. One can combat them in actual time by reacting slower and using breathing to anchor the situation. One can find positivity, identity, strength. One can programme one's mind to see the advantages in a situation, to find strategies for an illness or to just be more physiologically fit. I find it is important that I am acting not being acted upon by society and depression or psychosis. This incorporates not being swayed by others opinions but seeing outside yourself at your behaviour. One cannot see the woods for the trees.

This is often where CBT or NLP comes in. Rebellion is the spell that is caste in youth and is often extended into our 20's when we are caught in a void pocket. Friends warn you of not following president and the folly of non conformity- to still be in awe of authority when order proves to be wrong is folly in itself. When one opens a door there is a time lapse. A thinking moment when the future becomes the inevitable. Be decisive, create a market. Solve a problem many different ways- do not recognize failure. Don't apologise. Use your voice for good. Such it is when we accept or decide not to accept. There is something about this realization gap that is important. To conform or not to conform- which door to open? One can listen to Mozart after rock just as one has to learn to iron the shirts or do things for other people as a matter of course. The topsy-turvy Christ like view is here described. It is not what is behind the doors it is the choice. What would be good for you is often missed and can be overlooked. What could seem pointless can be essential. What could be disliked is something that is liked. Fitness is good for mind, body and soul. What could be unwanted may be something wanted. I once received a gift of a book when my sister got a china horse. I was so upset until I realised that the book was in fact better. Not showy or glitzy but useful.

Be comfortable with your own pain. Nothing very good or very bad lasts for very long. Part of maturity is not running to solve problems. Stay with it and it will usually subside. Shifting focus implies therefore shifting responsibility also implies authority not being in authority – a conflict. We need order to live peacefully. While we are post-Eden dwelling humans, we need order but we should embrace our humanness. Rejoice in what is laid out for us in the here and now. Like children, we want to learn our own way, we want to make mistakes and those mistakes may need to be made a few times for us to cognitively accept a change in the way we do things. The great thing about God is that we see concepts turned upside down- the outcast of society is the closer to God. Turn things on their heads. If you treat yourself too easily life will become difficult. If you procrastinate, problems will mount up. If only more people could see it that way, we may see a shift in how mental health is viewed. That vulnerable people going through major change are extra special and though they may seem weaker than weak they in fact have a will that is strong enough to change the world. I believe that most of the negative attributes of a person going through a realisation have been put upon them by society. We need to find our way out of the woods.

CBT gives credit to oneself vs Christianity, which gives credit to God. Without Christianity, CBT may cause a person to gain an inflated ego that comes with good self-esteem and confidence. Remembering that the wider picture is spiritual humbles the person into realising that we as humans don't have the answers to everything. Vole understood his CBT experience as providing him with a valuable neutral human contact and sounding board, as a link between psychiatrist and religion. Vital to vole as a fast-track tool in a society where it is not possible to drop everything to get better (i.e. go to a retreat), CBT provides quick, accessible, easy-to-use methods to change the way we think about a situation (the process of disowning the devil's view). Badger was a highly skilled therapist who understood the specific needs of a person who had suffered. When Vole was too unwell to even approach the church, it was

CBT that kick-started his ability to socialise. In hindsight vole believes that God was still the foundation; that it is ok to rely on therapies but that therapies alone are not the answer. This was a little confusing to understand as religion and CBT looked at how to maintain good human condition in different ways. Fear for example – face your fear – expose yourself regularly. (CBT) In Christianity, how do we cope with fear? By knowing that God is with you whatever and that through prayer, God's will for our lives is the path that we will tread through the forest of life.

The great thing about God is that he knows there is a time for everything and only he knows when that time is. He only changes us in ways we can accept. However much we may work on relieving anxiety through therapy, the time may not be right to let it go. It is very helpful to know how it is possible to let it go and to work with it by continually exposing oneself to fearful situations. By knowing that repeatedly doing so there was no harm done to vole in the process confirmed to vole that life was going to be okay. In order for Vole to leave distress behind, there had to be a mixture of 1) the shock of realisation settling time 2) an awareness of self-maturity confirmed through the actions and responses of others 3) time to get over the physical effects of the trauma.

Trust not in being judged by friends and society, nor in the cleverness of any that lives. Concentrate in the ticking of the clock. Do not look to others to rehabilitate you but take the major pillar of mindfulness: non-judging, patience, a beginners mind, trust, non-striving, acceptance and letting-go. The internal dialogue can then be calmed so that one is aware but just letting it be. Much of mindfulness practice is awareness of self, based on meditation and a useful example of this is tai chi or prayer. Psalm 143:5 states, *I remember the days of long ago; I meditate on all your works and consider what your hands have done.* Through self awareness of paying attention to your deepest self, we relinquish control by observing and accepting things as they are and not constantly trying to change things in the deluge of life- to have clarity, simplicity, security and prayer. Enjoy walking though the forest of life.

This acceptance of our thoughts and emotions can be perceived as living in the present moment and paying attention not in the past or the future, but in the here and now. In Matthew 6: 34 we are instructed by Jesus to *Give your attention to what God is doing right now, and don't get worked up about what may or may not happen tomorrow. God will help you deal with whatever hard things come up when the time comes.* Both the casting away of distraction and the need for a decisive break from the past are both spiritual and psychological compunctions. A certain man being in anxiety of mind, continually tossed about between hope and fear, and being on a certain day overwhelmed with grief, cast himself down in prayer before the altar in a church, and meditated within himself, saying, "Oh! If I but knew that I should still persevere," and presently heard within him a voice from God, "And if thou didst know it, what wouldst thou do? Do now what thou wouldst do then, and thou shalt be very secure." And straightway being comforted and strengthened, he committed himself to the will of God and the perturbation of spirit ceased; neither had he a mind any more to search curiously to know what should befall him hereafter, but studied rather to inquire what was the good and acceptable will of God, for if I'm honest the Lord consummates a fair few concepts like unconditional acceptance that I see in my daughter's eyes to win loyalty and nurture, which he would give gladly, responsibly and sweetly.

One can stimulate well-being by seeing the positives in anxiety. It is often the follow up process in therapy which leads to understanding, acceptance and hence to be able to think good thoughts again. *Finally, brothers, whatever is true, whatever is noble, whatever is right, whatever is pure, whatever is lovely, whatever is admirable--if anything is excellent or praiseworthy--think about such things.* Philippians 4:8. Illness is the surest way to make me think that heaven should fail but really I should be looking at the good aspects of it- the heightened awareness and humour. I am always brought back from the brink by the most stoic of characteristics- to keep a sense of humour, and see the absurdity of the situation, which is often in the detail:

A flock of fruits bobbed me by
I counted one to twenty five
The gutter's current was so strong
Is this where they all belong?

Some had advantage over others
In size and streamline shape
Eight berries disappeared in haste
Followed by a tireless grape

The long enduring banana boat
Saved four kiwis, entirely soaked
So away they did float

From what I could not say
To a filthy life of misery
To escape the master's appetite?
Soon out of sight, they'll be quite alright.

Next there came the apple race
A speedy cox would ne'er disgrace
With braeburn and gala close behind
And three pink ladies sweet and kind

Who upon stopping the melon ship
Came across a damson pip
The greengage said 'she fled the scene
For fear of being made unclean'
(She had eloped with nectarine
And couldn't face the tangerine)

I must have watched for many days
Their dancing, darting jamboree
But what to do in a reeking haze
Of vermin, germs and dysentery?

And then a cherry stopped to ask
Had I seen a banana pass?
I told him briefly the ordeal
And he looked at me with great appeal

He told me how he'd heard one case
Of a London chef who to his disgrace
Had ousted the finest, juiciest peach
Without a single bite to preach

So, unemployed and quite alone
That poor peach rolled from home to home
And gathering friends of similar heed
Planned the mightiest, dirtiest deed

Hence operation projectile punch
(Guaranteed to go down well with lunch)
Would spurt from every major sewer
No chemist would offer an effective cure

Absurdities! I shrieked aloud
And shut my eyes to the barmy crowd
I can't believe for one whole week
I've witnessed floating fruits that speak!

At last, I turned by back to leave

In doing so, I began to heave
'Revenge' I heard the cherry cry
As gruesome stench refused the sky.

Chapter 9 The Parachute of Faith

The fiend who did not understand the formation of the postcode has sparked off the dreadful hate of them again. I mean what is the bloody point? 688 instead of 6HH. When they get it right, instead of thinking them just normal, I am immediately pleased with them and view them as this kind of genius thing for getting it right and I am relieved. Normal people are just so infuriating. Just as one should not be singled out for praise for being wacky so one shouldn't be praised for normality. Society tends to reward normality and extroversion, while segregating distracted and introspective notions as strange and unhelpful. Mannerism, the powerhouse of the Renaissance; bizarre distortions of human perspective, should be the ideal. I live life with structure and the appearance of normality but one should not be any the less able to fathom, experiment, explore and so on. When convention fails us we are caused to explore the unnorm. It is an impertinent suggestion I realise like the rings in the tree and the knots in the wood I never really wanted anything from anybody. I fear normality. Normality stands in rows by verge, solitary silent, in penitence for their awakening. Nothing will lie there for each other in times of indecision like heaven's providence: and something has to come from nothing and nothing comes from something.

Normality has to include aspects of mental health and everyone has explorations into life unless they just accept rules and regulations. Only by broadening your mind can you conquer your fears. By differentiating beliefs and rules you can manage and prosper. Nevertheless most people are fragile to the outside world. Vulnerability, if we forget our public image is from these creaking glass cages. Fear keeps me from sleep, because of my shyness that I bolted like a fox from his den to fend for the vixen and his child for to roam. My daughter is fearful of the noise and bustle and I am helpless but to show a respectable indulgence to create understanding and happiness, showy and definite. I remember this hesitantly while composing over the virtues of the day. How can we teach our children to be sensitive when the world is so chaotic? Not until now have I returned the sentiment I kept it for far longer than was necessary, like a flower in a dusty bride's bedroom. I saw others acceptance and reflections of myself as overly important and hence got trapped in the expectations of society and my appearance to others. The rising of the fiery phoenix from the ashes has played a unique role in my pride, which was diminished by society.

I....
The boy jumped from his muse
I shall conceal the blame
Come, come to me
I have seen you at your worst
Spiteful and bitter sore
Will disappear if only you draw near
I....
The boy cast his eyes hither
I will bring you jewels in my arms
Sink, sink into me
I read you like a book
Adventures and pictures galore
Will come alive if only we contrive
I....
The boy stretched out his arm
I will devour your dreams
Glow, glow with me
I will throw you pearls of the past
The sacred core
Will sooth if only you move into the fire
I....

The boy reached into the flames
I will raise you like a phoenix
Rise, rise with me
I will glorify in my arms
The life you bore
Will last if only you are caste…

The phoenix from the flames is a way of delivering souls. It is from my Uncles ashes that I have risen. *It is vanity to love, that which quickly passes away, and not to hasten where eternal joy abides. Strive, therefore, to turn away thy heart from the love of the things that are seen, and to set it upon the things that are not seen. The grace of God. Be rooted in Jesus and you will bear abundant fruit. Do what lieth in thy power, and God will help thy good intent* (Imitation of Christ).

My journey through prayer to fulfilment is to be like a parachute, on the journey from the heaven of before and after*…. and witness Heaven, which thou thyself didst call to witness the promise thou hadst made me; and if all this fails, thy own conscience will not…* Heaven is up to you; if you keep those things made in life it will be yours forever like Don Quixote's promise. Knowledge persists throughout, waiting to be revealed by experience. One knows everything one needs to know and life is its discovery. Life was a chain of events over time and though the initial conditions may be changed. Trying was the meaning of life, belief the point. Jesus concluded that individuals could not control the outcome of destiny. Fundamentals had repercussions throughout time and these fundamentals could not change. The detail of the tapestry of life could be changed but whose patterns remained the same so that heaven is the destination when life's rich pageant is played out.

We have transfiguration when the memories, reverberated in those last moments of heightened awareness, raise the bridge of hope reaching even the immeasurable love in the realms of the infinite. It is so that Michael thought of no grander proof of the sovereign Lord. It is a feeling of serenity and peace engulfing, contradicting with the approach of a storm, and bringing the world gusting towards us containing letters, which we never meant to send. Freezing – the place, the attitudes, time.   Vole's sense of self had retracted or refracted? He headed toward the kitchen stumbling, bruising, and aching. He leant upon the sink and turning his head upwards to the right, he noticed a tunnel that was grey and ribbed inside (a little like a vacuum cleaner hose). This was no ordinary tunnel, as usually (vole had enough sense to draw this conclusion), a tunnel would diminish in size as it went into the distance.   This tunnel exploded the law of perspective. The further away it went, the larger the area inside, and in the uttermost distance was an image, so close and radiating power and trust, an image of the most amazing love in an expression that vole had never witnessed before. If vole had been asked to draw this image he may not have been able to for vole said "our faces say a lot about us" - imagine taking the love element written on the faces of our people and placing them in one image and knowing in an instant that that image emanated love and that that image draws close to comfort the wretched. Vole was consumed with love and knew that it was God. How long had it been? Vole did not know. Similar to a traumatic incident, time had slowed/distorted. However to the contrary, this was the most welcome event vole was to experience.   Time stood still, time was completely insignificant. Time did not exist. It didn't need to.

Vole was left standing alone. Strands that weaved the life he wanted became untied. Others were untying too.

The knot of faith pulled him through. The tapestry was then able to be weaved like the incident that started this whole saga. The demise of the *Mongoose*. In front of Michael; when he slipped through the sound barrier, but all around, was a huge space, dark but filled with a million lights "What you see is what you want," said a strange hallowed voice. The eternal meteor flew just to meet the sun again peeling back the night as time flew past. The sky's the limit to a limitless heaven whose plan guilds our waking lives to reason, guiding us through death upon conclusion? Where flight is the nerve tingling meaningful where treatment of life's mundane and fractious is forgotten in our repose, what is the purpose of our existence? The spark of constant memory is a demand for the truth of mystery, the opposite to sods law –a universal constant of the substitution principle of the universe- contained within God's words. *Father in heaven! It is from Thy hand that we receive all. Thou stretchest forth Thy powerful hand and it seizes the wise in their foolishness; Thou stretches forth Thy powerful hand and worlds pass away. Thou openest Thy compassionate hand and it fills with abundant blessing all that live, and if at times Thou seemest to take Thy hand from us, we know that Thou dost only close it in order to conceal a blessing yet more abundant. We know that Thou dost only close Thy hand in order to open it again and to fill abundantly with blessing all who live.* (Kierkegaard)

I wonder what the last musical sound will be. The ends of the earth. The apocryphal silence. The discord of elemental collapse perhaps, when rhythmic resonance, to the ear breaks the chord of intimacy the sound bears an incantation. True music of closeness. Or perhaps a slow peaceful exhalation of breath. A sigh. A crash, a cacophony of whispers. A deathly silence. There must be no sound in time. Time must have a stop at the speed of sound. In the depths of silence no words are needed, no language required. In the depth of silence I am called to listen. Listen to the movement of the spirit. "Be silent," saith the Lord "and know that I am God." At the end of the world there will be only two sounds- harmony and discord. The harmony of a final pause. The discord of dread.

A celestial hum followed, the gathering of angels. We found ourselves all at once surrounded by a host of dancing daffodils. They stood, feeling the breeze, the root tendrils making the ground shimmer between them and nature. The dark sods of earth beneath sustained its stillness. When soft daffodil, open to the virus breaks, the heir of intimacy sees as imitation the true art of closeness. They could not move, like the children in excitement, like children they watched from its still vantage place as it stretched, never realising but promising spring. The delicate lines of its petals broke the air like a bell resounding, like a sole survivor of a great flood, proud and in many ways unsubstantial in the daybreak. Its colours were leant by the sun, its smell by the fairies. It was a cup of its own liquor, almost drunk on its realisation of life.

Life was short, life was fulfilling. It had a span, which dealt in moments, not months or days. It was a focal point to the children who passed it, who asked inquisitively of its youth or colour. It was a statue of its own beauty. A so enticing miracle of spring standing still. Thickly remembering *hallelujah* out on the parade ground: regimentation was charm in the world of the solitary daffodil to the host surrounding. Then came the angels, yonder breaking from the form of the daffodil; the communication of intimacy as the soul alights revelation of the true grace of closeness with God. In life it was a small bubble of air 'neath a pillow of dreams. It was the open suitcase at the start of a holiday, the heady excitement of the pleasure of freedom. It was the stare of a girl, the meditative swirl, and the antics of a horse running because he wants to. The foothold in virtue. It was the look of a child sitting content. It was the content of a Chinese takeaway. The taking away of pain, the replenishment of life. The affirmation of a kiss, the consequences of a wish. It was everything and nothing, the spark of recognition, the suppliance of a thought, the exhilaration of flight. It was to be in the palm of God. *May the road rise up to meet you. May the wind be always at your back. May the sun always shine warm on your face; the rains fall soft upon your fields and until we meet again, may God hold you in the palm of his hand* (Irish proverb). In death I will not fear. With it I will not find fault. With it I will not search for self. With it I will glorify my support. I will just let it be in the palm of God.

The very cherubs huddled all together, like birds when soars the falcon and they felt a tingling to the tip of every feather and formed a circle like Orion's Belt around these poor charges of many coloured flame, until its tinges reached the speck of earth and made new aurora borealis spread its fringes. ©Byron The motion of time played in their wings and they shone like the glare from the sun in a mirror so that one could not comprehend their features but one could feel their love and compassion from their voices which valued and gave triumphant feelings to them. The cherubs expressed choices to us, testing but feeling their way into our inner calm and serenity. He felt them lift him up and show him what his life was worth and it arose to the bridge of hope reaching even the immeasurable love in the realms of the infinite. As we looked into mystery it was a childhood scene, a statue, the hustled adulation of a crowd, the peace of a country village, the dismay of missing someone; but overriding it all, a feeling of fulfilment in a moment of truth until he was floating on hope and fear. He was a statue forever, ripples of cognitive behavioural boundaries and Christian emotion emanating from, and washing over him, spread like the development of purpose so that heaven would be glorified and conviction found.

He stood like a statue
Chained to his devotion
Communing with God
Composing nature
Consumed by winter
Pounding upon her grave expression
Martyr bound
Like faithful praise
Incidental
Praise found
Like a winter bourne vision
Her head bowed in passion's gaze
For prayer became
Spirit in movement
The last fantastic place
Between a man and a woman
A statue of virtue
Amongst anxious worlds

We felt at one with our surroundings, consumed and emanating from ourselves and the feeling of another, closer than fiction, was the mystery of cherished moments exploding from pinnacles of light. The space between the candle and the flame. The sense of female energy engulfed us and we felt like being caressed by a hundred warming hands massaging the pressures, limits and spiritual wants we harboured. Our achievements were beauty, and beauty knowledge, so that all creation was suddenly known which captured the universe like the summer loving we had known as teenagers. A rose fanned out in front of us. Amazing to sit next to this rose, through heaven we know that the present is forever and time is a convention. Knowledge persists throughout to be revealed. We know everything we need to know and life is its discovery. We can only wonder and learn to be content and care for ourselves in a way that God does. If wonderful works were easily translated by human reason they would not be wonderful. By knowing God's love we can join our hopes and alleviate our fears:

Until he said I love you
I was as a chrysalis
Fermenting in the ether
A wanton shadow
Chasing pleasures
Putting rainbows on wedges of cheese
Looking into the rose of love
And eating from the goblet of man
The final word was spoken
With such reticence that
My heart bellowed its memory
Time was of no importance
Dreams were a threat
Though ebbing moons
Would ever shine this way
Bewildering
Its soft caress comforting
Distance- friend and enemy
Launched its wing firmly through
The night kindled there
Blankets never heavy enough.
Clutching
This emptiness sustaining

I never thought I was much good at prayer but then I realised that I had been praying all along with the connection to my uncle. Whatever hope exists hold on to it like a parachute for it is only through hope that the sound barrier can be broken. It is up to us through prayer and petition to glorify heaven. The idea of heaven is there if you act upon it. Figures are growing around the world who have the strength to bring people to salvation. This surrounds the idea of being born again. The phoenix was an Egyptian myth from the spiritual primitive. To me it suggests that you may have to go to hell and back to find out the truth. Hence mental health. The resurrection brought us to the meaning of afterlife and if we follow Jesus our place in his father's house is assured.

Does psychosis in fact take on a form of possession or mental health issue? The book shows the positivity in trying and that spectral diversity and the subtleties between illusion and illumination is actually belief...I think the book has illustrated that this space between the candle and the flame is perceptably holy and nothing is impossible with God. *O Lord you have searched me and you know me. You know when I sit and when I rise; you perceive my thoughts from afar. You discern my going out and my lying down; you are familiar with all my ways. Before a word is on my tongue you know it completely, O Lord. You hem me in- behind and before; you have laid your hand upon me* (psalm 139). We must still learn to break the barrier between man and God. To travel as fast as sound seems the perfect psychosis. This doesn't mean that just because He cannot love us more or less than He does we should just accept heaven. No we must fight the good fight to ensure that it does not fail. What if heaven should fail is a warcry to fighter pilots to do their duty. Our insignia to bring the gospel to society.

The Tree house looked so cosy that night, not dissimilar to that which Christopher Robin visited on occasion. And it was an occasion that night.

'Vole, where are you?' exclaimed owl. Vole sat slightly reclined in his port stained armchair. His eyes seemed to be looking towards a lamp on an oak stand. Owl looked into his eyes yet they gave no meaning that owl could relate. Owl looked down to see that vole was clutching a scroll in his hand. Owl stooped to take it from vole's cold hand. As he unravelled it, he saw words and equations that owl felt equated to the meaning of life.

Owl knelt down next to vole and placed his hands on voles lap. He turned his own head toward the lamp. Mumford and Sons played in the distance.

We walked away from the house and as we turned to look at its tired brick and decayed wooden creaks, a warm pain rose in my heart and my throat was sore with a charge of teary contemplation.

I looked through the lit window and a shadow of the two creatures resided on the yellowed wall. Hence came vole and owl, hands held toward the empathy of the clouds on a sunny morn. The river's flow was crisp and clear. Ten fish jumped effortlessly. The bees rivalled the roses and time was allowed to stand still for just a little while so that we could acknowledge the beauty of life. We were born to love, all its wonders to know. To travel as fast as sound seems the perfect means to understand creation. I have done this through listening and quiet petition to an uncle who seemed to have the perfect answer. The meaning of the word *belief*. That we were made to meet our maker with the beauty of discovery, and that magic that was lost a long time ago was ours, not tied to an old stone grave, but in heaven.

Lightning Source UK Ltd.
Milton Keynes UK
UKOW050747211211

184169UK00001B/2/P

9 781849 916899